NURSING EDUCATION IN A CHANGING SOCIETY

T0317396

Published on the occasion of the fiftieth anniversary

of the University of Toronto School of Nursing

Nursing education in a changing society

EDITED BY MARY Q. INNIS

University of Toronto Press

©University of Toronto Press 1970
Reprinted in paperback 2017
ISBN 978-0-8020-1697-3 (cloth)
ISBN 978-0-8020-6112-6 (paper)

Contributors

Helen M. Carpenter, R.N., B.S., M.P.H., ED.D.
Professor and Director, University of Toronto School of Nursing

Blanche Duncanson, R.N., B.S.N.
Associate Professor, University of Toronto School of Nursing
Director, Nightingale School of Nursing, Toronto

Oswald Hall, B.A., M.A., PH.D.
Professor, Department of Sociology, University of Toronto

John D. Hamilton, M.D., F.R.C.P.(c), D.S.
Vice President, Health Sciences, University of Toronto

Dorothy J. Kergin, R.N., B.S.N., M.P.H., PH.D.
Associate Professor and Associate Director, School of Nursing,
McMaster University

M. Kathleen King, R.N., B.A., B.S.N., M.S.N.
Professor and Associate Director, University of Toronto School of
Nursing

Jean C. Leask, R.N., B.A., M.A.
Director in Chief, Victorian Order of Nurses for Canada

Helen K. Mussallem, R.N., B.S.N., M.A., ED.D., LL.D., S.D.
Executive Director, Canadian Nurses' Association

Kathleen M. Parker, R.N., B.S.N.
Instructor, Atkinson School of Nursing, Toronto Western Hospital

Ronald R. Priest, B.S.
Chairman, Liberal Studies Department, Mohawk College of
Applied Arts and Technology, Hamilton

Dorothy G. Riddell, R.N., B.S., M.A.
Assistant Professor, University of Toronto School of Nursing

Marjorie G. Russell, R.N., Certificate of Nursing Education,
University of Toronto School of Nursing
Formerly, Nursing Consultant, Department of Veterans' Affairs,
Ottawa

J. D. Wallace, M.D., F.A.C.H.A.
Executive Director, Toronto General Hospital

Morley A. R. Young, M.D.C.M., F.R.C.S.(c), F.A.C.S., F.A.C.H.A.
Medical Superintendent, Archer Hospital
Administrator, Lamont-Smoky Lake Auxiliary Hospital

Contents

Foreword

It is fitting that in the celebrations of the Fiftieth Anniversary of the founding of the School of Nursing of the University of Toronto an attempt should be made to record certain of the salient features of the School itself and of its influence upon the broader interests of education for nursing throughout this country and beyond. This book reflects the interpretation of the term nursing education as conceived by the founder, pointing out, and rightly so, that progress has been made in the general setting of a rapidly changing society, which includes the changing status of women.

Within this general context, the book has given effective emphasis to two principles held strongly throughout the School's life, namely, that in progressive nursing at all levels the preventive and the curative go hand in hand and that those concerned with the preparation of the nursing team should recognize the need for sound education not only at the university level but for the diploma student and the nursing assistant also. Purposeful effort has been directed to the actual practice of these concepts in a variety of ways throughout the past five decades.

The School has served during a period when nursing has been emerging as a full-fledged profession. The interpretation of the needs of nursing education has been fraught with difficulties from both within and without the profession. Many of these were encountered by Miss Russell, the founder of the School, who, had she been lacking in conviction and importunity, might easily have been defeated.

On the other hand, the book reveals that, from the establishment of the former Department of Public Health Nursing until recent years, the School has been blessed with friends of insight and distinction; among these are a former Director of the School of Hygiene of the University of Toronto, Dr. J. G. Fitzgerald, and Dr. C. J. O.

Hastings and Miss Eunice H. Dyke, formerly Medical Officer of
Health and the Director of Public Health Nursing of the Depart-
ment of Public Health of the City of Toronto, respectively, and Miss
Jean I. Gunn, a former Superintendent of Nurses of the Toronto
General Hospital. Claiming honoured mention is the name of Dr.
H. J. Cody, a former President of the University of Toronto, who
at a critical stage determined the future usefulness of the School.
It has been noted that the Canadian Red Cross Society and the
Rockefeller and Kellogg Foundations have played significant roles
in the School's life, thus contributing in a marked fashion to nurs-
ing education in this country and in the international field as well.

All will agree that the indispensable factor in the achievements of
the School was its great good fortune in having had Kathleen Russell
at the helm as Director; a brilliant leader who, combining the vision
of the idealist with the action of the realist, succeeded in founding
a school, the guiding principles of which are destined to outlast an
era of pronounced social change. Methods will undergo adaptation
to meet the changing needs of society, but the educational principles
enunciated by Miss Russell will stand the test of time. Not only did
she hold these beliefs with conviction but she inculcated in others
the professional faith which she herself held so strongly. Thus, as
the years moved on, there was gathered around her a carefully selected group of staff members who accepted these principles and
with dedicated ability, each in her own specialized area, contributed
immeasurably to the total strength of the School. Through combined
effort in a pioneer field there has emerged a remarkable degree of
co-operation with and acceptance of departmental units within the
University on the part of community health and hospital services.

The reader will welcome comments on the future of health services
and the education of nurses in meeting new community needs. Already, significant progress has been made in stabilizing baccalaureate
degree courses and in planning for graduate work which, it is expected, will be offered in the fall of 1970. Those who were intimately
aware of Miss Russell's goals for the School possess an abiding faith
in its present and future direction and in the part succeeding graduates will play as members of the staff and alumni. Ours is a rich legacy of mind and spirit, which will continue to lend inspiration and
guidance to those responsible for the School's welfare in the present
and throughout the decades to come.

Florence H. M. Emory

Preface

A fiftieth anniversary calls for celebration and few forms of celebration are as wide-reaching and long-lasting as a book. The present volume commemorates the founding in 1920 of the School of Nursing of the University of Toronto. However, the book has a much broader scope than the history of the school and its founder. Doctors and nurses from many branches of their professions present here their experiences, views and prophecies. Naturally, each expresses only his own opinion. Combined they give a wide-scale picture of Canadian nursing education as it adapts itself to a time of rapid social change. It was thought fitting to end the volume with an essay by a post-basic nursing student who looks far into the future in which she will play a part.

A generous gift from a graduate of the class of 1921, the late Mrs. Atholia L. Cherry (née Beatty), has made possible the publication of this book and is here gratefully acknowledged. We also gratefully acknowledge a grant from the Varsity Fund for the publication of this book.

Mary Q. Innis

PART ONE THE EMERGING PROFESSION: 1920–1970

1
Social change, specialization, and science: Where does nursing stand?

OSWALD HALL

Today there are very few occupations whose practitioners are not concerned about their present status or anxious about their future. The pace of change in the world threatens to make even the well-established occupations obsolete; it also exposes them to a struggle against new competitors. Nursing in Canada is no exception; over the past decade its members have become highly sensitized to the hazards of living in a changing society.

An attempt to understand what is happening to the profession of nursing leads one deep into the study of a whole society. In a profound sense nursing is one of the oldest and most fundamental of social activities. It reflects the fact that one human being – usually a woman – can care about, and care for, another in his hours of helpless need, yet without becoming too deeply involved emotionally. Yet, although nursing carries the imprint of a very ancient and essential occupation, it also reflects a modern world in which vast numbers of new occupations are beckoning to women and are inviting them to see themselves first and foremost as parts of the work world and only secondarily as mothers and homemakers.

The study of nursing also brings one face-to-face with the foremost aspect of our society, i.e., its technological character. Ours is a society based on science and on the technical uses to which science can be put. Nursing and medical care reflect this fact. The care of the sick in our society now involves an immense array of specialized workers each with his own kingdom of scientific knowledge and his own armament of technical expertise. These have been brought together, housed, supported, and organized in the hospital. To study nursing in its natural habitat is to study this great modern work institution with its vast numbers of employees, its almost infinitely fine division of labour, its oft-times incredible machines, and its capacity to transform all these into a going concern.

A study of nursing is, therefore, essentially a study of the fundamental features of a society; more particularly of the place of women in the social system, of the variety of specialized occupations that have emerged in the society, and of the kinds of specialized institutions within which work is done.

THE CHANGING OCCUPATIONAL STATUS
OF WOMEN IN MODERN SOCIETY

It is commonplace in this decade to deplore the shortage of nurses in Canada. The apparent unreadiness of women to devote themselves to a career in nursing is anomalous, to say the least. It is not a field in which men compete vigorously or devise barriers to exclude women. It is an occupation with an established and respectable reputation, in which girls of any class level can feel comfortable. Moreover the shortages occur even while progressively larger numbers of women are finding their way into the working world. Why don't more working women choose nursing as a career?

It seems clear that the number of women entering the nursing profession is influenced by social changes which initially may seem remote. One of these is the increasing participation of women in the work force. In 1921 approximately 20 per cent of Canadian women were employed. By 1960 this figure had climbed to 30 per cent, a figure that is still somewhat low beside US levels, but large enough to call seriously into question the notion of the Canadian woman as mainly a homemaker. The trend has gone on relentlessly, slowly but cumulatively.

The increasing proportion of women participating in the work force is to be noted at many levels. More women now have full-time jobs as opposed to part-time work. The increase occurs regardless of marital status. However, one of the more surprising findings is that the married women are marching into employment at a faster rate than are either of the other two groups. For example, the proportion of married women working in Canada almost doubled in the decade from 1951 to 1961. Of course, married women form the largest category of all women, and an increase among them affects the total proportionately, but it is among them that the swing to employment is most marked and most consequential.

This change in the readiness of married women to seek employment is parallelled by adjustments they have made to family life. Several of these are worth noting. First is the tendency for girls to marry earlier; the age of first marriage for Canadian girls has slowly been going down. Accompanying this change is the tendency for women to have the first child at an earlier age. Her reproductive cycle starts earlier than formerly. Moreover, the number of "higher-order" births has decreased to a conspicuous degree. The decline in the Canadian birth-rate, which continues on into this decade, is very much a matter of a reduction of "higher-order" births. In other words we have moved to a pattern of two- and three-child families, with a vast reduction in the number of large families.

What is most impressive, however, is not the reduced size of families, but the fact that the actual child-bearing period has been remarkably compressed. In other words, not only are women having their last child at a very early age, but their child-bearing cycle has been significantly shortened. As a consequence, their child-rearing cycle also has been shortened markedly. In effect this means that, in general, women in Canada are being liberated from their historic tasks of bearing and rearing children, and as a consequence are finding themselves with an extended "post-family" period in their lives, unlike anything ever experienced before by Canadian women.

In the light of these changes we can readily understand why more women are participating in the labour force. Most single girls and young married women try their hands at employment, perhaps to give it up once family responsibilities become substantial. Then, once the children are launched on their own lives, the married woman is freed to come back into employment. Hence arises the so-called "twin-peak" pattern of employment. Women aged 20–25 are very heavily represented in the working world, whereas those 25–35 are not. The women aged 40–45 are again heavily represented.

We can see in these matters the ways in which two social changes combine and eventually reinforce one another. A change in the way families are organized creates the conditions that permit women to return to or remain employed. But the opportunities for employment encourage women to complete their families early. In both these matters Canadian women are following a trail which has been blazed by their sisters to the south. The two changes are continent-wide, and not merely Canada-wide.

One can also detect similar connections between the increasing proportion of women at work and the opening up of educational opportunities for women. It seems that education affects both of the matters discussed above. The more education a woman receives, the less likely is she to bear children in her later years. And the more education she receives the more likely is she to be found in employment as she reaches her middle years. The statistics on university-educated women bear this out with admirable clarity. For them, a very large proportion (about 45 per cent) are employed during their early years, i.e., 20–25, and, although half of these give up their work during the child-bearing period, a very high proportion (35 per cent) come back into employment after rearing their families. In their case it is fairly clear that all three social changes, i.e., family pattern, increased education, and employment, are interrelated in a way that mutually reinforces these changes.

THE VAST ENLARGEMENT OF SPECIALIZED OCCUPATIONS

The world of work into which women move is now dotted with a myriad of distinctively specialized occupations. The emergence of ever-larger numbers of occupations has helped create new social strains. Few parents can discuss with their children, with any degree of authority, more than a small handful of the new occupations that have arisen in the past decade. Moreover, the members of occupational groups find it progressively difficult to comprehend what goes on in neighbouring occupations. As the number of occupations increases it becomes ever more difficult for young people to make ready and rational decisions about their life work; it also becomes progressively difficult for occupational groups to launch effective campaigns to attract new recruits to themselves in appropriate numbers.

This trend toward specialization in work is not easy to grasp in its full extent. The Canadian Census does not attempt to count and report the full range of occupations in our society. It limits itself to reporting *classes* of occupations. Even these general classes are relatively numerous. The census volumes use approximately 250 classes to encompass the range of individual occupations that are reported. Since each of the classes mentioned above may include a hundred or so specific occupations, the total number of occupations is formidably large.

The first large-scale effort to count occupations on this continent was carried out about thirty-five years ago and resulted in the publication of the *Dictionary of Occupational Titles*. At that time there were in existence about 23,000 different occupational titles, of which at least two-thirds represented specifically identified and distinctive occupations. Since then the number has continued to grow.

This massive growth of numbers of occupations rests largely upon two other developments in our society. These are the growth of scientific endeavours and the utilization of scientific knowledge in technological pursuits. If there is a growing edge to the field of occupations, it lies along the line where science and technology are meeting. Each of the sciences is itself not only growing but tending to subdivide. Each of the highly technical occupations is tending to split up into new fragments that later may emerge as occupations in their own right.

The Department of Manpower in Ottawa has attempted to document the variety of occupations arising in this field of professionals and technologists; the results are arresting. Sociology, a rather recent arrival among the sciences, has over forty sub-branches. Psychology has still more, and economics more again. The subfields in the biological and physical sciences now surpass the hundred mark. In the technological field the engineers have experienced a comparable expansion. Not too long ago there were four types of engineering – civil, electrical, mechanical, and mining. Now there are over a hundred distinctive branches recognized and listed. In brief, the very special class of occupations called "professional and technical" has in a brief span of time subdivided into over a thousand specific occupations.

The world of specialized occupations, however, is not divided symmetrically between men and women, particularly those professional and near-professional occupations that one might usefully compare with nursing. Among them one finds instead a high degree of differentiation into men's work and women's work.

In a very broad sense the world of work is, of course, a man's world. Most men spend their whole adult lives in it, whereas only a minority of women do. But, as noted above, this is changing. Roughly

30 per cent of women in the age groups likely to supply workers are actually engaged in employment. Hence, in general, one might expect to find about three times as many men as women in any of the various fields of employment. Of course, for many occupations, like logging or mining, the work could scarcely be handled by women. But the fields where masculine strength and stamina are essential are now few and marginal. Most occupations require an ability to use ideas, or words, or to tend relatively delicate machines, and in all these fields one might expect men and women to be represented in the same proportion as that in which they enter the labour force. But the facts are quite otherwise. In the old established professions, law and theology, women rarely appear. According to the 1961 Census, only one lawyer in forty is a woman. Among the clergy the figure is one in sixty. In the newer professional fields a similar condition has developed. Only one engineer in approximately four hundred is a woman. Engineering in Canada is man's work.

In health, one is faced, by contrast, with much greater participation of women. Indeed, here women outnumber men, two to one, in the whole field. One could say, therefore, that women are greatly over-represented, since in employment in general they are outnumbered three to one by men. But this more equal participation in the healing professions is more apparent than real. Among the ancient professions of physicians and surgeons, one finds only one woman for every twelve men. Among more recent specialties in the healing field, the proportion is still less. Among optometrists one finds one woman for every thirty men; among dentists the ratio is one to twenty.

But such imbalances also occur in the opposite direction. In nursing it is the women who outnumber the men. Here one finds only one man reported in the census for every twenty-five graduate nurses reported in employment. In training institutions for nursing one finds one man for every seventy women in training. In other words, women are represented there 200 times more frequently than would be expected, given the general level of employment of women. Nursing is an overwhelmingly feminine occupation to much the same degree that engineering is a masculine occupation.

There is a distinct pattern in the clustering of each sex; the men seem to predominate where science and expert technology are aspects of the occupation, whereas Canadian women, if they do not shun these, are found in occupations little influenced so far by science and technical expertise. In the larger world of work, one area to which women have flocked in large numbers is that of clerical employment. There was a time when a clerk was a strictly masculine figure, but today the field is heavily feminine. There are five women for every three men in this area in Canada. This is the sector where women have penetrated most deeply into the modern corporation, and seem destined to displace men even more substantially.

By contrast, women play a very small role in managing and directing business concerns of any sort. They work as secretaries and clerks for the managers, but scarcely compete with men for the managerial jobs. There is only one woman engaged in any sort of managerial role in Canada for each eight men so employed. Men organize and manage our large work organizations, whereas women fit into these in a very different set of work roles.

Nursing, however, has not shared in the burgeoning subdivision so characteristic of the general world of work; indeed, nursing seems to have striven hard to maintain its traditional forms in the face of the fantastic growth of new medical occupations round about them in their daily work.

THE DIVISION OF LABOUR IN LARGE WORK ENTERPRISES

In turning attention to the kinds of places in which work is done we are focusing on another major facet of modern society. Ours is a society of large-scale organizations, a world of bureaucracies, of establishments, of corporations, of huge institutions, to use a few of the substitute terms we use when the reality becomes monotonous. The extent to which life in this century has taken on this quality can scarcely be exaggerated. We are "organizational" men, parts of an "employee" society, members of an "industrial" state. We open our eyes first in a large maternity ward, spend our school and university years in large educational institutions, gain our incomes from large business corporations, buy our food and clothing from large retail establishments, travel by large transport systems, end our lives in a large hospital, are prepared for burial in a mass mortuary, and are sent on our way by the spiritual representatives of a large religious institution, leaving our estates (small rather than large) to be handled by the large tax department of a large government.

There was a time when the only really large institution encountered by the ordinary citizen was the military establishment. But eventually armies needed factories to provide their weapons. These early work organizations bore many of the features of army life, in terms of their patterns of discipline and their modes of supervision. But soon the factory system took on a life of its own; and as the factory became the chief means of producing goods, its organizational form was transferred to other fields of work, especially those that provide services. We are currently the heirs of an organizational revolution through which most of the basic work activities of life are now carried on in large-scale institutions. And as a corollary most of us, in our daily work roles, spend our lives in one or more of these large organizations. This, of course, has befallen nursing; the work of the nurse is very much that of the employee carried on either in a massive hospital, or in a smaller one that apes the larger models.

But in comparing the hospital to the factory, and to its predecessor the army, it is important to recognize two special features which in a sense set the hospital in the forefront of organizational change in our society: science and technology. Anyone trying to write a history of hospitals would be confronted by a mass of other changes. At one time the hospital was largely the house of death. Later it turned into a temple of hope. More recently it has become in effect one of the public utilities to be supported by the state and available to all. The hospital has been at the vortex of swiftly moving changes.

Enmeshed in the various changes impinging on the hospital, though, are two that require elaboration. The first involves the amassing of scientific and technologically sophisticated personnel in the organization. These hordes of workers are part and parcel of most work organizations. There is hardly any kind of work that does not depend on the scientist and the highly trained professional for its welfare. But what is distinctive about the hospital is the predominance of such people among those who work there. Whereas in most industries the highly trained personnel may constitute a small segment of the total, and perhaps one isolated from the main activities, in the hospital the main working figures are the highly trained professionals. They put their imprint on the organization; indeed, one might say that the hospital more and more takes its character from this central corps of professional workers.

The influence of professionals on the nature of the hospital shows up most vividly in the matter of supervision and control. Professionals are extremely difficult people to control in work situations. In their case the time-tested procedures of military life, in which one person issues commands and another obeys, seem totally out of place, as do the available modifications of such control devices. The reasons that those who practise the historic professions are difficult to control are not really difficult to fathom. Such people are the custodians of specialized scientific knowledge. In their efforts to apply such knowledge it is necessary that they respond first and foremost through their personal store of scientific knowledge, something that cannot be mediated by a second person. A second requirement of such workers is their capacity to exercise responsible judgment in the application of their scientific knowledge, that is, to hold themselves responsible for the consequences of the procedures they undertake or even of the advice they provide to clients. In work situations of this sort a professional can ill afford to put himself under the orders of another, since this would interfere seriously with his own exercise of judgment.

The second notable feature of the hospital is the amassing of technological equipment. In part this is an aspect of the growth of science, although once scientific knowledge is built into a machine it no longer requires the scientist to operate the machine. The hospital is now very much the locale of a vast array of machines of great variety and complexity. The omnipresence of the technical equipment gives to the hospital a distinctive character. Those who work among the machines must take on, to some degree, a facility for such a way of life. That is to say, they must feel at home in the daily running of the machines, in their repair when they falter, and in the imaginative adaptation of the machines to new functions. As one can readily envisage, this feature of hospital organization creates the need for a vast pool of workers to man such machines. These workers must be specialized to the requirements of each type of technical equipment; and they also must be specialized further in terms of whether they tend the machine, or merely monitor it, put it to rights, or devise improvements on it.

This two-fold character of hospital organization poses two very cogent problems for the nursing profession. How far has nursing moved in the direction of accepting science, scientific effort, and the implications of science as basic features of the nursing enterprise?

Have nurses embraced the developing technology of medical care, or held it at arm's length, or indeed rejected it as incongruent with the tasks of their field?

As to the first of these it seems clear that, to date, nurses have not tried seriously to focus their work efforts in a scientific mould. While medical care has been specializing along new types of diagnosis and treatment at a bizarre speed, nursing has shown no such trend. It has devised no bodies of knowledge concerning the nursing function comparable to what surgery or anaesthesia have contrived in their efforts to modify the functions they perform and the goals they pursue. This is not to say that nurses are anti-scientific. What they seem to be doing in this area is largely to borrow the scientific apparatus of related occupations, and, moreover, to restrict themselves to dealing with the problems of some other field of work than their own. Many of their efforts at scientific research seem more like fragments of medicine than aspects of the nursing enterprise. There is nothing inherently wrong with such efforts in the direction of science; the point is that they fail to focus directly on nursing matters, thereby to bring nursing into the framework of scientific effort in an emphatic way.

The forays in the direction of medical research do not exhaust the scientific endeavours of nurses. They have expended considerable effort and resources in the work of the social sciences and the behavioural sciences. What seems lacking in these efforts is again a direct attack on nursing phenomena by the use of the tools of these sciences. Here, as in medical research, nurses have largely been content to discipline themselves to carry out some of the scientific tasks of psychology or sociology as additions to their expertise as nurses. But so far they have not translated their own work into the idiom of social science so that their problems can be tackled from a fresh perspective. In short, nursing seems to have allied itself to the great movement in science only in a halting and limited way. The impact of science on nursing and on nurses has been tangential rather than direct and is still barely perceptible.

When we turn to the relation of nursing to technological developments, the picture is more complicated. The advent of the technological revolution in the hospital has been marked by the emergence of an immense number of new tasks and a veritable army of occupations of very recent origin. Some of these are the modest tasks of machine tending, some are more like skilled trades, some smack of supervisory and organizational skills, and others lie on the fringe where new scientific knowledge is subtly being transformed into new technological advances.

These technological developments in hospital life are visible in many directions, but can be grasped most readily by focusing on the technical laboratories and on the technicians and technologists who work in them. In a very brief period of time these have specialized, in a twofold sense. The laboratories have themselves become specialized so that in a modern hospital there may be at least five distinctly different laboratories with different functions, different techniques, and different personnel requirements. Furthermore, within each of the laboratories the process of specialization is underway, giving rise to a significant number of distinctive occupations in each laboratory. In a recent study for the Committee of the Healing Arts of Ontario some forty different kinds of occupations were discovered in the hospital laboratories.

The arresting fact about this development is the almost total absence of nurses from such patterns of growth. Nursing has not extended its domain to incorporate these new growth and new emerging tasks in the healing enterprise. The initiative has come almost totally from other segments of the system. Neither have they individually sought a place under the new umbrella of exciting specialized occupations that has emerged. Instead they have remained within their older sphere, even though these new developments have offered much in the way of power, prestige, and income to those entering the new occupations. The exceptions are the nurses who function in the clinical-investigation units or the intensive-care units. But in these they play a role very subordinate to the medical personnel on the scene.

On balance it seems that nursing has stood aside from both these two great changes impinging on our society, both of which are exemplified so dramatically in the very hospitals in which the work of nurses in now predominantly carried on. As a result, it is other occupations, once extremely modest and inconspicuous, that are developing bodies of knowledge, special expertise, and control over expensive equipment, and are thereby gaining access to income, power, and prestige in the healing field.

One can only speculate as to the forces acting on nurses to prevent them from venturing into these challenging areas of the healing enterprise, into the main streams of change affecting their work. The reasons seem to be twofold. One goes back to the division of labour by gender. In medicine it was the men who early came to occupy the autonomous positions where power, knowledge, prestige, and income were at their peaks, whereas women were allocated the lowly tasks where service to others, control by others, and deference to others were characteristic of the job to be done. What evolved in medicine on this continent was in effect a castelike structure, with men ordained to one sort of work and women to another sort. These caste structures are everywhere formidably resistant to change, since each part comes to accept as natural the relative power of the other. Neither doctors nor nurses have demonstrated a readiness to change their relative statuses in healing.

The other set of forces that has inhibited nurses from competing for the newly emerging jobs in medicine is of a more subtle sort. Although doctors have relegated nurses to a lowly share of the work of healing they have also granted them, in chivalrous fashion, a share in their own prestige. Nurses have traditionally been second-in-command in the healing enterprise. And even if being second in a group of two means being at the bottom of the scale there is some balm in considering oneself only second from the top. This way of looking at things has prevented nurses from changing substantially their tasks in the healing field. Because they have felt assured of the number-two spot in the realm of hospital organization they have paid scant attention to what the newly arrived occupations were achieving in terms of technical proficiency and a distinctive body of scientific knowledge. But sooner or later the newer occupations take on technical functions and their technical specialization opens the way for them to become autonomous to an increasing degree. It is just their technical importance and increasing autonomy that now places the field of nursing in a disadvantaged light. Nurses have tried to hold their ground while the other occupations have been occupying new terrain.

While the newer paramedical occupations have been jostling for a place in the hospital system, something has been happening in the general area of hospital organization. Doctors have traditionally been in the top positions in the medical enterprise, with nurses next in line. However, as hospitals have become larger, and particularly as they have become more complex, doctors have tended to renounce the position of chief administrator. Few doctors now view the position of hospital administrator as one that confers high prestige. Their renunciation of these positions has been paralleled by the emergence of a whole new set of functionaries, the professional hospital administrators. It is worth noting here that nurses have not emerged to occupy these new centres of power that the doctors have vacated. Hence, we have the anomalous situation that, although doctors tend to treat nurses as second in command, those in command in the hospitals are neither doctors nor nurses but a new breed of professionals. The power position of nurses must now be seen in its relation to these new central figures of power and authority. What seems to be happening at the moment is the proliferation of administrative officials in the hospital system with nurses very largely relegated to one department in a system of many, many departments.

As noted at the beginning, nursing in common with a host of other occupations is beset with problems clamouring for attention. There is concern over recruitment, over training procedures and facilities, over conditions of employment, over styles of union organization. Many of these matters reflect the fact that nursing is irretrievably involved in the basic changes impinging on modern society. Nurses are inescapably caught up in large-scale organizations, since there are almost no other ways in which they can put their skills to use. They are inexorably caught up in the competition of new occupations in the healing field. They labour in a field where scientific knowledge is increasing by leaps and bounds, and the urge to apply it technically grows relentlessly. With these basic trends of change nursing has a rendezvous.

2
Nursing and the law:
The history of legislation in Ontario

DOROTHY G. RIDDELL

The Province of Ontario has been chosen for study here because it has the largest number of nurses and the control of its legislation has been delegated to each of three types of registration authorities. Also, it is the province the author knows best.

The development of nursing in Ontario covers almost a hundred years – 1872 to the present – with 1922 marking the date of the first legislation, an Act respecting the Registration of Nurses. The fifty years prior to 1922 marked a new era in hospital management, and one in which trained nurses and training schools were essential features. In this period, too, although some twenty years after the training schools were established, nursing began to emerge as a profession organized primarily to combat the rapid increase in the number of training schools and to improve standards of nursing education. The years since 1922 have been a time of continuous effort on the part of the profession, and, more particularly, on the parts of those nurses responsible for the development and implementation of legislation.

1872–1922

Nursing[1] as a public secular entity began in Ontario during the years 1872–96. Accomplishments in social welfare and industrial and technological expansion allowed people to turn their attention to various kinds of practical humanitarian work. It was natural for women to go to the hospitals to care for the sick at the bedside.

Until 1872, hospitals[2] received financial assistance from the provincial government without any reference to the work being done, other sources of income, or the inspection of institutions. But in 1872[3] the government began to inspect hospitals and benevolent institutions and to require a report on the buildings and systems of management. Under the Charity Aid Act,[4] 1874 (in force until 1912), hospitals no longer needed to exist as public charities for the sick and indigent because a more equitable method of distributing grants of money was found. Thus, with public recognition, financial aid, and supervision, many improvements were made and the hospitals increased and expanded.

Nursing was then one of a number of services that came under the supervision of the Inspector of Prisons, Asylums, and Public Charities, among whose duties[5] was the inspection of hospitals. Reports depict the origin of training schools for nurses and the importance of the work of the lady superintendents. On nursing in one hospital the inspector wrote: "A most commendable feature in the management of this hospital is the superiority of the nursing service – It would be well if other hospitals would adopt the same means of training nurses instead of putting up with incapable and inexperienced persons."[6]

The inspector pointed out the unlimited opportunities in nursing and Canada's great need for trained nurses. Because of this need, hospitals both large and small opened training schools. In 1883 there were three hospitals[7] with training facilities, and by 1923 at least one hundred were in operation, all of which varied in size and standards. Most of the nursing care was given by the pupils in training for there were few "trained" nurses on the hospital wards. The lady superintendent was in charge of the hospital and the training of nurses. About one lady superintendent, the inspector said, "This lady performs all the duties which require in some other hospitals a medical superintendent, a matron and a steward, and having regard to the quantity and quality of work done, this institution stands in efficiency second to none in the Province."[8]

The inspector worked extensively with the mental institutions. It was important to him that they should be considered as hospitals and that standards should be set for the cure of patients. He placed strong emphasis on the quality of staff. In the report of 1879, the inspector referred to "the kind and intelligent men and women in constant attendance upon insane people – closely observing their habits and practices, looking carefully after their wants and keeping them employed, interested, and amused."[9] Training schools for nurses were subsequently opened in the larger mental institutions.

This proliferation of training schools and the lack of nursing standards worried the lady superintendents for they wanted their pupils, many of whom would go to the United States, to have successful careers. The loss of nurses from Canada to the United States was a matter of concern to the medical profession. Sir William Osler reported in an address to the Canadian Club in Toronto that the number of nurses who had migrated from Canada to the six great hospitals on the Atlantic seaboard was one-third of the total of 651 trained nurses employed there.[10]

The lady superintendents saw the need to organize hospital and nursing services in order to give better care to the sick. As pioneers in a new field of nursing they had the capacity for hard work and thoroughness. In entering the realm of social welfare they were influenced, no doubt, by women such as Florence Nightingale. To the lady superintendents and to the religious nursing sisters, the people of Ontario are indebted, for it was they who gave an essential service in the provision of patient care and at the same time formalized the traditional concepts of nursing into a practical humanitarian service for a young and growing country. Two ideas emerged at this stage of nursing evolution that were to influence the type of legislation to be enacted in later years. One was the generally accepted idea that the apprenticeship system of training nurses was satisfactory and economical; the other was that institutions receiving public financial support must come under government supervision.

As the lady superintendents worked to improve nursing conditions in the local hospitals, other Canadian nurses were destined to a prominent place in a new movement to reform nursing. Historically, the opportunity to participate in nursing affairs came through the educational and employment opportunities which the United States offered liberal-minded Canadians at the end of the nineteenth century. Three young women who went to the United States to train as nurses were, among others, to initiate a new movement for "organization and legislation"[11] as a way to improve nursing. Two of the Canadian-born women were Miss Isabel Hampton (later Robb) and Miss Mary Adelaide Nutting. Although they remained in the United States, they were interested in Canada and saw that Canadian nurses had an opportunity to share in developments taking place in the United States. The third person, Miss Mary Agnes

Snively, who trained "for the express purpose of fitting herself for a hospital position in her native land,"[12] returned to Ontario to be Superintendent of Nurses at the Toronto General Hospital in 1884. According to Roberts,[13] Miss Snively had "a concept of nursing reform in Canada" and she became an acknowledged leader in Canada and other countries.

The World's Fair in Chicago, 1893, marks the time and place of the new women's movement to reform nursing. Eighteen superintendents of leading training schools in the United States and Canada met under the chairmanship of Miss Hampton at the Hospital, Dispensaries, and Nursing Section of the International Congress of Charities, Corrections, and Philanthropy held in Chicago at that time. Influenced by Mrs. Bedford Fenwick, President of the British Nurses' Association, and an advocate of legal control by registration of nurses, the women decided to form a Society for Superintendents of Training Schools in United States and Canada. The new society was organized in 1894, and its purpose was promoted with the slogan "organization is the power of the age, without it nothing great is accomplished."[14]

With this challenge, the number of nurses' organizations increased rapidly at local, provincial, state, and national levels. The International Council of Nurses was organized in 1899. The history of these organizations is complex, but reference is made to one for its influence in the development of nursing in this province, the Graduate Nurses' Association of Ontario, established in 1904 and incorporated in 1908. It was a voluntary organization the aim of which was to advance educational standards in nursing, to maintain the honour and standing of the profession, and to further necessary legislation in the interests of the public, the physician, and the nurse.[15]

As the movement for organization and legislation gathered momentum, it was inevitable that there would be opposition and delay. Hospitals, particularly the small ones, feared that their training schools would be closed. The very thought of an organized group of women caused apprehension to some. Occasionally, nurses objected if they felt their livelihood threatened, and, to a few, the movement directed toward the elevation of standards of nursing education was a denial of the emphasis that should be placed on standards of nursing practice.

In Britain, Miss Florence Nightingale opposed registration of nurses, although Woodham-Smith[16] reported that her objections were not so much to the idea of registration itself as to the kind of registration proposed at that time. To Miss Nightingale, qualifications by examination did not take into consideration the character training which she held to be most important. In her opinion, nursing was "too young, too unorganized and contained divergences too great for a standard to be applied."[17] Abel-Smith,[18] in reference to Miss Nightingale's objections, stated that she thought reform should come about by example rather than by regulation.

Meanwhile, at home, the National Council of Women of Canada[19] supported the movement for nursing reform. It was natural that the National Council should assist the nurses, for it stood for equal educational, industrial, professional, and political rights for women. The Council of Women held to the idea of adequate and uniform registration acts in the provinces and the reorganization of nursing education. It assisted the Graduate Nurses' Association of Ontario to present its first proposal for registration to the legislature in 1906.

Superintendents of training schools in their communities allied themselves with women's and nurses' organizations and at the same time they took on the self-imposed task of interpreting the needs of nursing to their hospital boards. What was accomplished in the local situation was due largely to their insight into the situation at hand and their ability to effect change.

In Canada, it took some twenty years before every province obtained nursing legislation. Nova Scotia was the first to enact registration for nurses in 1910, and Ontario was the last of the nine provinces. (Newfoundland, prior to becoming a province of Canada, obtained registration in 1931.) Throughout, the nursing profession viewed legislation as a means of overcoming an overwhelming problem; registration was the means to an end, not an end in itself. To a number of individuals, however, registration of nurses was not the most effective means of controlling nursing education. In 1914, a Canadian nurse made this perceptive statement: "Registration at its best is merely a bolstering up of a system which is radically wrong, and no satisfactory plan can be evolved until the training of nurses is put on a sound educative basis."[20]

In Ontario, the opposition and delay that the nurses met had to do with two policies observed in public administration: one, the protection of the public against the possibility of monopoly by a profession; the other, the delegation of legislated responsibility. The issue that was to develop in the efforts of the Graduate Nurses' Association to obtain registration, was whether a voluntary organization of nurses could obtain the legal authority to administer a system of registration for all nurses. A brief description of events surrounding the efforts of the Graduate Nurses' Association to obtain legislation in 1906, the reading of Bill 106, an Act respecting the Graduate Nurses' Association, is given here, not to suggest the lively times associated with the enactment of legislation, but rather to indicate how policies may be viewed differently by the people concerned, such as nurses, physicians, legislators, hospital authorities, and visitors from another country.

The *American Journal of Nursing* describes the views of two American visitors, Mrs. Isabel Hampton Robb and Miss Sophie Palmer, who attended a meeting of nurses and legislators to discuss the implications of the proposed bill for registration. Mrs. Robb had been invited to this meeting to explain developments in the registration movement in the United States. Mrs. Robb took exception to one clause in the bill which dealt with the composition of a council to administer the legislation, for not all the members were to be nurses. In her opinion the control of the profession should be in the hands of nurses only. Miss Palmer, who was with Mrs. Robb primarily to inspect training schools of Ontario for the New York State Education Department so that their graduates might register in New York, objected to the clause restricting membership of the council to British subjects resident in Ontario. Miss Palmer thought this clause unfair to nurses of other countries who might be residing in Ontario. To her, registration was an educational measure, not a political one.

The editor[21] of the *American Journal of Nursing*, in reporting on the visit of Mrs. Robb and Miss Palmer to Toronto, wrote:

... We are inclined to think that at least a few of the Canadian Nurses have lost sight of the fact that registration is not a local measure, that it is a broad professional movement, that the standards set in one state or country affect the nurses in every other state or country, and that in the framing of such laws every effort should be made to have the essential points as nearly uniform as possible, that reciprocity between states and countries can eventually be entered into without having to tear down or reconstruct.

There are many nurses of the broader liberal type in Canada, but they are in the minority in the registration movement, and those who are leading would seem to be too much under the dominance of outside influence.

In the liberal group we think may be found nearly all the Canadian women trained in the United States who have returned to Canada, and the superintendents of training schools as far as we know them. We hope that the criticisms made by Mrs. Robb, a noted Canadian living in the United States, and Miss Palmer, who is one of the American leaders in the registration movement, may at least set the conservative party thinking. In a women's movement based on educational principles there should be no attitude of exclusiveness shown between states or countries.

At the first reading of Bill 106, the Graduate Nurses' Association had asked, once incorporated, to administer a form of compulsory membership which would affect all nurses employed in hospitals. However, at the second reading of the bill the request was modified to mean registration of graduates of organized courses. In reporting the discussion of the bill, a newspaper said, "The gallery of the legislative chambers was crowded yesterday afternoon and evening by nurses and their lady friends who are interested in the bill respecting the Ontario Graduate Nurses' Association – The ladies followed with visible eagerness the discussion on the measure."[22] The paper outlined changes that were proposed in discussion of the bill and concluded the afternoon's report with, "It seems to be assured that most of these suggestions will be embodied as amendments and carried."[23]

When a special committee met to discuss the proposed changes, the members were unable to promote the bill further and subsequently the Graduate Nurses' Association asked that it be withdrawn. The specific reasons for the defeat of Bill 106 are not clear. Generally it was supported, although the government was not committed one way or another. One legislator said he "was in favour of it but not as a close corporation. It was reasonable that every care should be taken to protect the public – the objection came from those who did not understand it."[24]

The failure to obtain the authority to administer a system of registration was a great disappointment to the nurses and their friends. Although they did not present another bill to the legislature until 1922, the intervening years were not lost, for the profession had time to strengthen its position and to gain additional support from colleagues and friends.

During these sixteen years the publication of two reports on medical education was to influence profoundly the development of nursing. The first report by Abraham Flexner[25] on medical education in the United States and Canada brought about widespread changes. Flexner prescribed criteria for admission to medical schools and standards for development of the curriculum. He also emphasized the importance of clinical teaching. The results of his recommendations were that many medical schools were closed. In reference to Flexner's report, Macfarlane[26] points out that "These changes were incidental to the new movement to convert medical education from apprentice training given largely by practitioners to the new concept of its being a full-fledged university discipline."

Because the findings of this report were applicable to nursing education, they served as guidelines in the changes that were to take place in the nursing schools. Obviously, apprenticeship as it was in the preceding century could no longer be the acceptable method of educating nurses.

The second publication, the *Report of the Royal Commission on Medical Education in Ontario*, dealt directly with nursing and other occupational groups as well as medicine. At this time, 1917,[27] there were 2200 nurses resident in Ontario and 61 hospitals, some of which were very small. Altogether, 400 pupil nurses graduated each year. The report brought out the need for "uniform preliminary educational qualifications, standardized comprehensive professional training with outside inspection and strict examinations."[28] The report proposed that registration provide for more than one category of nurse as well as for those in special work; and that a Council of Nurse Education be appointed. The Graduate Nurses' Association was commended for its work in obtaining better standards for correlating the programmes of the various training schools. The report advised that registration be administered under the existing statutes and that nurses have a voice in nursing matters.

Although government had taken its initial step in legislation for nurses by inserting Clause 18 in the Hospitals and Charitable Institutions Act, 1912 (in effect until 1930),[29] for the registration of graduate nurses, regulations were not implemented since not all hospitals with training schools came under the authority of this Act.

Clause 18 was subsequently revoked when the Act respecting the Registration of Nurses was passed in 1922, this time without dissent. The authority to administer the new Act was invested in the office of the Provincial Secretary, not the professional association.

An inspector of training schools, a nurse, was appointed by the Provincial Secretary, in 1923. When the authority to administer the Act was transferred to a new Department of Health in 1924, a newly appointed inspector assumed responsibility for the Nurses' Registration Division in that department.

In developing a system of registration, Ontario was influenced by New York State,[30] which had enacted nursing legislation, with provision for an inspector, twenty years before. It was apparent that the State Board of Nurse Examiners of the Department of Education in Albany recognized the importance of the right kind of inspectional service, one that would give scope in developing educational programmes, advise superintendents of nurses, and represent government in nursing affairs.

The Graduate Nurses' Association viewed the Nurses Registration Act as a compromise, for it had sought the authority to administer the legislation. The Association acknowledged that the government might have fewer enforcement difficulties at first, but said it had not achieved the legal status it hoped for. To the Association "the opposition did not seem to be to registration as such but to the granting of legal status to nurses founded on the principle of self-government and to the setting up of standards which could compel many hospitals to either close their schools or meet the standards."[31]

The struggle of an emerging profession of women in the early years of the twentieth century is part of the larger problem of the status of women. The enactment of nursing legislation was a reflection of the general improvement in the position of women in Ontario when they received in 1917, as an acknowledgment of their contribution to Canada's war effort, the right to vote.

1922–1962

A new era in nursing in Ontario began with the enactment of nursing legislation and the incorporation of the Registered Nurses'

Association of Ontario in 1925[32] (formerly the Graduate Nurses' Association).

In the new profession, the public began to see the registered nurse as a professional person who carried heavy responsibilities, and the less well trained practical nurse as one who had important work to do. Nurses were employed in public and private hospitals, sanatoria, and mental institutions. They also worked as practitioners or "special nurses" in private homes. With the expansion in public health services and advances in medicine, nurses began to move into wider occupational horizons as public health and visiting nurses, teachers of nurses, supervisors, and administrators in hospitals both at home and abroad. As they moved into these new fields, they saw that extended preparation was needed; consequently, nurses and employers turned to the universities for help. As a result, the first course in teaching and administration was offered by the Extension Department of the University of Toronto in 1928 with an initial enrolment of twenty-one students. Other certificate courses of one academic year followed. Shorter "postgraduate" courses in clinical nursing were given by a number of the larger hospitals as a means of obtaining qualified personnel.

Enactment of Legislation

Since 1922, five acts and their amendments have been enacted. Under each act there are numerous rules or regulations to indicate how the act will be implemented and by whom it will be administered. Regulations undergo change as new situations arise; they are deleted when they are no longer useful; or they remain unchanged under a new act. In this way, regulations provide for both continuity and constant change. Approval of the Lieutenant Governor-in-Council is required to enact a new regulation. By this means government retains a measure of control of the legislated responsibility it delegates to a registration authority.

Regulations affecting nursing represent minimum standards, a base line, above which each school of nursing can set its own requirements. Consequently, regulations reflect, not the ceiling of attainment that schools actually reach, but rather a floor below which they may not fall.

Registration is a system that has become an accepted means of distinguishing between the "qualified" and the "unqualified"[33] for two categories of nurses, the registered nurse and, later, the registered nursing assistant. In Ontario, these two legal categories represent the profession. Government has delegated responsibility to three types of registration authorities since 1922, the Ontario Department of Health, the Registered Nurses' Association of Ontario, and the College of Nurses of Ontario, a statutory body to administer the Nurses' Act, 1961–62.

As each act has changed, and with it the regulations, the nursing profession has moved closer to its goal of being self-governing; that is, to administer its affairs and to formulate rules and policies. A summary of acts, Amendments to Acts and Regulations, given below, should reflect a philosophy of legislation as well as the more specific detail of restrictions and privileges which affect basic nursing education. Although this digest attempts to identify major regulations, it does not show their continuity from one act to the next or when they were deleted. For the exact interpretation of the acts and regulations, the reader should refer to the Ontario statutes

Only brief reference is made to the nursing assistant in this chapter.

(1) An Act Respecting the Registration of Nurses, 1922
(Nurses' Registration Act) and Its Amendments of 1929, 1933,
1937, and 1944

This Act provided for the establishment of a training school in a hospital, sanatorium, sanitarium, and, under the amendment of 1933, a university. Graduate nurses in Ontario and those registered elsewhere were entitled to registration by waiver of examination for a limited period of time and only those who registered were qualified to use the title of registered nurse. No one was barred from earning a livelihood. Provision was made for the appointment of persons to administer the act and its regulations. The amendment of the act in 1929 relating to payment of a fee; the amendment in 1937 prohibited persons from conducting a training school without authorization; and the amendment in 1944 provided for a director of the Nurses' Registration Division and staff, and postgraduate courses of instruction.

The regulations under the Act permitted an institution to conduct a training school provided that minimum requirements in the various

branches of nursing were offered, or were arranged through an affiliated course in another hospital, the conditions of which were to be
outlined by the inspector of training schools. Approved training
schools were to offer at least two years of general training in one or
more hospitals that met requirements.

Examinations based on the provincial minimum curriculum were
arranged in designated centres throughout the province at least once
a year. Each candidate for examination was required to be a graduate of an approved training school, a resident of Ontario, of good
moral character, and twenty-one years of age. A nurse graduated
from outside Ontario could sit for examination under certain requirements. Each registrant received an initial certificate of registration, and an annual certificate of renewal. Revocation and suspension of registration for fraudulence was provided for.

The minimum staff in the hospital consisted of the superintendent
of nurses, an assistant superintendent, and a night supervisor, all of
whom were to be registered nurses. The superintendent of nurses
could be superintendent of the hospital.

Although the essentials for residence and classroom equipment
in the training schools were outlined in regulations as being desirable, the hospital or institution was required to provide a recreation
room, adequate lavatory facilities, and single beds for night nurses
in a quiet section of the hospital.

The training school was required to keep records of instruction,
and, as far as possible, students were to be admitted in classes. They
were to have two years of high school or a satisfactory substitute on
admission to the training school. The hours of "duty" were not to
exceed fifty-eight per week and all time lost was to be made up. A
preliminary course of not more than three months was necessary before allowing students to assume nurses' responsibilities. Transfer
of students from one school to another was approved by the inspector, or the Council of Nurse Education, so that on completion of
the course prescribed they would be eligible for registration. Although it was desirable that students have some experience in "special duty" in homes for periods of time under two months, the fees
were not to be collected by the hospital for such services.

A Council of Nurse Education was appointed in accordance with
regulations, and consisted of seven members, three of whom were
connected in a teaching capacity with a training school and were

recommended by the Registered Nurses' Association of Ontario; two were physicians; the inspector of public hospitals and the inspector of training schools were *ex officio* members. The council was to advise on regulations, examinations, the affiliation of students in other hospitals, and standard record forms, and it was to receive reports brought to it by the inspector.

The first regulations set forth in 1929 by the Ontario government outline the time to be spent in theory and hospital services as shown in Table 1.

Regulations of 1944 prescribed the duties of the director of the Nurses' Registration Division. The director, appointed by the Lieutenant Governor-in-Council, was responsible to the Minister of Health. Her duties related to the enforcement of regulations, conduct of examinations, and maintenance of a register. She could assume the duties of the inspector, as required. An inspector was appointed with duties prescribed by regulations.

Examinations, the portal of admission to registration and the profession, were required of all graduates of approved schools of nursing in Ontario. Examination papers were written in both French and English. Registered nurses from countries that met Ontario standards could register without examination. Canadians living outside Canada unable to register for reasons of citizenship could register in Ontario by examination.

Regulations relating to suspension and revocation of registration applied to those guilty of malpractice, those convicted of criminal offence associated with nursing, those mentally and physically incapable of the practice of nursing, and those who were incapable of nursing because of alcoholism or use of drugs.

The conditions under which a training school could be conducted were specified. Each superintendent of a training school filed an annual report of the activities of the school and at the same time made application for renewal of approval of the school. The names of all students admitted were submitted in writing to the director of the Nurses' Registration Division. The length of the course was three years. The admission requirement to the sixty-four schools of nursing was increased to three years of high school, and after 1944 the Secondary School Graduation Diploma (four years of high school) was the minimum requirement for admission to the profession. Students were required to present birth certificates showing that they were at least eighteen years of age.

The membership of the Council of Nurse Education increased to not more than nine persons. *Ex officio* members were the Deputy Minister of Health and the director of the Nurses' Registration Division. Other members included the inspector of public hospitals, a

---

TABLE 1

Regulations for the Conduct of Training Schools, Pursuant to The Registration of Nurses Act, 1922

Subjects	Minimum time
Theory	
Nursing principles and methods*	110 hours
Charting	2 hours
Dietetics†	24 hours
Hospital housekeeping	3 hours
History of nursing and ethics	6 hours
Bacteriology	5 hours
Chemistry	10 hours
Urinalysis	4 hours
Hygiene and sanitation	6 hours
Anatomy and physiology	32 hours
Materia medica	25 hours
Medicine	
General	10 hours
Contagious diseases	4 hours
Tuberculosis	6 hours
Venereal diseases	6 hours
Mental diseases	4 hours
Diseases of the skin	2 hours
Children's diseases (including infant feeding)	6 hours
Surgery	
General	8 hours
Orthopaedic	4 hours
Gynaecological	4 hours
Eye, ear, nose, and throat	4 hours
Obstetrics	12 hours
Hospital Services	
Medical nursing	3 months
Surgical nursing	3 months
Nursing of children	2 months
Obstetric nursing (including assistance at delivery of 10 cases)	2 months
Contagious-disease nursing‡	2 months
Mental-disease nursing (if possible)	2 months
Tuberculosis nursing (if possible)	2 months
Operating room	2 months
Holidays	1 month

*To as great an extent as possible by practical demonstration.
†To include instruction and practice in diet kitchen.
‡Scarlet fever and diphtheria services compulsory where and when possible.

physician teaching in an approved training school and appointed by the Registered Nurses' Association of Ontario, an officer of the Department of Education, and four (later six) nurses appointed by the Registered Nurses' Association of Ontario, one of whom was to represent the university schools of nursing. The Council had powers to make recommendations to the Minister for the better carrying out of the Act.

(2) The Nurses' Act, 1947, and Its Amendments of 1950 and 1951

This Act established a new category of nurse, the certified nursing assistant. It provided for the registration and protection of title of these nurses.

The regulations under this Act outlined procedures for the administration of the Act, and the registration, conduct, and inspection of training centres for nursing assistants and schools of nursing. One or more inspectors were to make required visits and submit reports of their visits. The duties of the director were prescribed.

Approved schools of nursing were asked to employ two nurse-instructors, and every department of the hospital where students were assigned was required to have a supervisor who was a registered nurse. Detailed requirements were included in the regulations for classrooms, residences, and teaching facilities. These stated that, in addition to the basic clinical instruction, schools were to arrange for courses of not less than eight weeks, and not more than nine, in communicable diseases and tuberculosis nursing. Subjects of instruction and clinical experience were now grouped into broad areas, that is, sciences, health and social education, and nursing and medical instruction. Theory and practice in paediatric and psychiatric nursing were to become effective in 1950–51.

(3) The Nurses' Registration Act, 1951 and its Amendments of 1957, 1961–62

This Act and its amendments authorized the Registered Nurses' Association of Ontario to administer the Nurses' Registration Act in respect to protection of title, registration, examination, discipline, admission to schools of nursing, and the curriculum leading to registration of nurses. It did not provide for the establishment, maintenance, conduct, and supervision of schools of nursing. The Act was administered by the Board of Directors of the Association.

Regulations provided for students to be admitted to schools of nursing at seventeen years of age and to present evidence of having taken prescribed science courses during their high-school years. Graduates of approved schools and courses who had not registered before 1926 had an opportunity to register without examination for a limited period of time.

The theory and practice as required in Schedules 1 and 2 of the Regulations are shown in Tables 2 and 3.

TABLE 2
Regulations Under The Nurses Registration Act, 1951: Schedule 1

Subject	Time in weeks
Medical nursing and nutrition in relation to nursing	30
Operating-room nursing and surgical nursing	30
Obstetrical nursing	12
Paediatric nursing	12

TABLE 3
Regulations Under The Nurses Registration Act, 1951: Schedule 2

Subject	Topics	Time in hours
Science	Anatomy and physiology	80
	Bacteriology	25
	Chemistry	20
	Nutrition in health and disease	45
	Pharmacology and therapeutics	40
	Psychology	10
Health and social education	Physical and mental health, the principles of teaching, and community health and social needs of the community	70
Ethics and developments in nursing	Ethics, history, development, and trends	40
Elementary nursing	Elementary principles and practice of nursing	150
Advanced nursing	Medical nursing	40
	Surgical nursing	35
	Obstetrical and gynaecological nursing	35
	Paediatric nursing	20
	Ophthalmological and otolaryngological nursing	15
	Nursing in communicable disease	20
Medical instruction	Medicine	20
	Surgery	20
	Obstetrics and gynaecology	20
	Paediatrics	15
	Communicable diseases	10

*(4) The Nursing Act, 1951, and Its Amendments of 1957,
1960–61, 1961–62*

This Act and its amendments authorized the Ontario Department
of Health to approve and inspect schools of nursing and training
centres for nursing assistants, and to register nursing assistants. The
amendments dealt with licensing and supervision of nurses' regis-
tries, the registration of persons trained outside of Ontario to register as nursing assistants, and the sale of courses in practical nursing.

Regulations during these years were specific and detailed in order
to legislate for that which may have been implied before, for example, the listing of equipment in the teaching area. In order to support the work of directors of schools and to promote community
interest, the regulations provided for advisory committees to schools
of nursing. Directors now had the privilege of attending meetings of
the hospital board when matters affecting the school were under discussion. Directors were required to have had a course of one academic year in a university in teaching and supervision. Two new
schools of nursing offering courses of two years were approved:
the Metropolitan School of Nursing, Windsor, and the Nightingale
School of Nursing, Toronto. The regulations were such that the already established schools of nursing could modify their programmes
within the three-year period to provide a final year of internship.

A survey[34] of hospital experience of student nurses based on an
analysis of certain aspects of the clinical field carried out in fifty-
four hospitals that conducted schools of nursing led to requirements[35] to control the amount of nursing service given by students
in hospitals, and to obtain facts which would be some indication of
the quality of service offered by each hospital in those areas where
students were assigned.

Regulations established a Council of Nursing with ten appointed
members, in addition to the Deputy Minister of Health and the Director of the Nursing Branch. The members included a representative of the Hospital Services Commission of Ontario; an officer of
the Department of Education; three registered nurses designated by
the Minister, who were directors of schools, of whom one was Director of a school conducted by a university; a duly qualified medical
practitioner designated by the Minister; two registered nurses recommended by the Registered Nurses' Association of Ontario; a member

of the Ontario Medical Association, recommended by that association; and a member of the Ontario Hospital Association, recommended by that association.

(5) The Nurses' Act 1961–62 and Its Amendments 1962–63, 1964, 1965

The Nurses' Act (a combination of the four previous acts) provides
for the establishment of a statutory body, the College of Nurses of
Ontario.* A Council of the College administers the Act. Members
of the Council are elected by and from registered nurses living in
twelve electoral regions in the province. Four registered nurses are
appointed by the Registered Nurses' Association of Ontario to represent the organized profession. One registered nursing assistant is
appointed by the Ontario Association of Registered Nursing Assistants to represent that organization. The Minister of Health, or his
designate, is an *ex officio* member.

The Act establishes two statutory committees, a Disciplinary
Committee and an Educational Advisory Committee composed of
five members from the Council, the Registered Nurses' Association
of Ontario, and university nursing education; and five members of
the Ontario Hospital Services Commission, the Ontario Hospital
Association, and representatives of medical undergraduate education. This Committee advises the Council in matters of basic nursing
education and the regulations pertaining thereto.

Regulations under the Nurses' Act apply to both schools of nursing and centres for nursing assistants. Schedules 2 and 3 outlining
the curriculum are designed to give each school of nursing the utmost
freedom in developing its programme.

Implementation of Regulations

Implementation of legislation, more specifically, regulations, is part
of an upward spiralling process which begins with a general acknowledgment on the part of the people concerned that a change in
the statutes is desirable and necessary. The timing of new legislation
is important, for, in order to effect change, it must be possible for
most of the people affected to meet its requirements. In general, a

* For clarification of the functions of the College of Nurses and the
Registered Nurses' Association of Ontario, see Registered Nurses' Association of Ontario, *The Professional Nurse in Ontario* (Toronto, 1968), p. 4.

new regulation must not be so minimal that little effort is required to implement or maintain it. Other factors related to timing are important too, such as the ease and speed of communication between people, and the urgency for legislation to be enacted. The Director of Nursing has an important role in arriving at a decision as to the appropriateness of action or inaction, and conveying her thoughts to the registration authority. The preparation and writing of proposals for enactment is the work of the registration authority with the participation of professional nurses in committees or as members of a board. This is a time-consuming task, which usually goes through several prolonged stages. Once legislation is enacted, a period of implementation begins. Implementation is most effective when it becomes a co-operative venture between the staff of the registration authority and the persons involved, that is, the director of the school, the staff, and the board of the school. Inspectors recognize that change is best brought about where there is conviction on the parts of all that change is necessary, and that more is to be gained through processes of consultation than through enforcement. Following the active period of implementation of legislation, a more or less lengthy and quiescent period ensues. When these particular regulations are no longer useful, they undergo further change, either by refinement to attain a greater measure of quality, or by elimination. Another spiral begins when the field is appraised anew to ascertain again the need for law enforcement.

It is to the period of implementation of legislation in the development of nursing in Ontario during the years 1922–62 that we now turn to identify phases of growth and discernible peaks of achievement. The three phases of growth extended roughly from 1922–31, a pioneering period; 1932–46, when standards were implemented and consolidated; and 1947–62, when standards were further refined and educational horizons were broadened through experimentation and innovation. It is less easy to specify achievements, for they can be ascertained only in relation to other historical events in the perspective of time. What has been achieved throughout is marked by the fine balance between flexibility and control.

The principles and practices of the central registration authority were for forty years affected by economic depression, war, epidemics, and expansion of health services. The number of active public general hospitals, most or many of which conducted training schools, continued to increase. In 1922 there were 101; by 1962,

177. To implement such a system, the registration authority worked at the provincial and national levels with people in many organizations, agencies, government offices, and universities. For example, the annual report for 1946 shows that the director and inspector worked in committees with the Ontario Red Cross and the Registered Nurses' Association of Ontario, the Department of Education, the University of Toronto School of Nursing, and the Canadian Nurses' Association. To the directors of nursing, the Nurses' Registration Division served, in the absence of a consultative service, somewhat as a clearing house for varied and many problems. Later, from 1955–59, it surveyed the need for, and subsequently established, a consultative service for hospitals on a voluntary basis.

The departmental reports and studies in which the staff of the Nurses' Registration Division participated provided background for legislation or for the resolution of problems.The wide range of topics has historical interest for they dealt with such matters as the cost to a hospital of conducting a training school, enrolment and withdrawal of students, numbers of personnel in hospitals, management of nurseries for the newborn, and the need for teachers.

In keeping with departmental policy, the professional association participated in preparing legislation and other matters. In the early years, it sometimes happened that the same nurses were members of the Council of Nurse Education, leaders in the professional association, and directors of schools, where they carried out the policies and regulations they helped to formulate. Specific matters were later dealt with through a joint committee arrangement, such as:

(*a*) A joint committee of representatives of the Council of Nurse Education and an equal number of persons from the legislation committee of the Registered Nurses' Association of Ontario was appointed in 1936 to study the revision of regulations for the registration of nurses and conduct of schools.

(*b*) A joint committee was called in 1938 to consider the advisability of offering a course for practical nurses.

(*c*) A composite committee of the Council of Nurse Education, representatives of the Registered Nurses' Association of Ontario, and the University of Toronto School of Nursing, was appointed by the Minister of Health in 1944 to prepare a plan for a central school to meet the need of a particular community.

(*d*) The Council of Nurse Education and executive of the Registered Nurses' Association of Ontario in 1946 prepared a statement on nursing education in regard to the cost of nursing the patient in a hospital, the proper organization of a school of nursing and the cost of operating it, and the need to increase the number of qualified teaching staff.

(e) A joint committee appointed in 1947 developed regulations for certified nursing assistants as required by the Nurses' Act.

The first pioneering effort (1923–31) provided a sound basis for registration and provincial examinations. (By 1927 there were 10,067 registered nurses with an annual admission of 1100 nurses to the register.) An inspection service for 110 training schools was instituted and the first minimum curriculum[36] was published. Following the development of essential criteria on which to base requirements, regulations were enacted in 1929. The annual reports of the Ontario Department of Health depict the scope and magnitude of the work accomplished by the inspector, who later became director of the division.

The work began with a survey[37] to obtain factual information. A programme of supervision was started almost at once, which directed attention to the improvement of nursing skills, the betterment of working and living conditions, and steps to safeguard the health of the student. As basic problems were resolved, assessment of clinical data for teaching and courses of study came under consideration. Arrangements were made for certain schools to affiliate with hospitals and for students to have supplementary experience so that all would be eligible for registration.

The second phase (1932–46), as indicated above, was one of implementation of standards, partly to limit the number of nurses graduating. Statistical data from annual and other reports of each school enabled the registration authority to establish criteria from which to work. The inspector, on the advice of the Council of Nurse Education, obtained[38] specific data on the schools. When the information was assembled, the schools were classified as approved (63, but all were not approved for living conditions), non-approved (9), and closed (28, but all of the hospitals continued to function). Other schools closed voluntarily at a later date.

This was the only time that schools of nursing were classified. The use of undue external regulatory controls seems to have been avoided, presumably to allow schools to develop from their own initiative. A similar policy seems to have applied to the size of hospital required to conduct a school, for rather than impose a rule as to the minimum number of beds it must have, the inspector left it for the hospital to show that it could meet the provincial minimum requirements and financially afford to do so.

The work of the Nurses' Registration Division was characterized by regular and frequent visits to the schools, meetings with hospital boards, and periodic conferences with the hospital and school staffs. (An example of the latter were the conferences held in twenty-eight hospital schools in which the University of Toronto School of Nursing assisted with collecting material.) At each visit the inspector directed her attention to observance of regulations in respect to students' working hours, the health service, admission requirements, the environment for learning, available clinical experience, and the course of studies including ward teaching. The importance of an adequate number of qualified teachers, the status of the student, and the school as an educational entity were basic considerations.

The proposed curriculum of the Canadian Nurses' Association[39] was a guide used extensively by all schools in a crucial phase of curriculum development. Following the Second World War, the second provincial curriculum was published.[40] It outlined minimum requirements, and for the first time provided essential information for the conduct of schools of nursing. This curriculum was modified and later used by the Registered Nurses' Association of Ontario until a new one was drafted, prior to the establishment of the College of Nurses of Ontario.

The period (1947–62) began with the need for additional personnel and facilities for the expanding health services, and the postwar growth in population. To meet the need for more qualified personnel, the province offered financial assistance to nurses to enrol in courses in teaching at a university for one academic year. The National Health Grants which have been given annually for study at a university (and several conferences for directors of schools of nursing) have been a stimulus to nursing education, for not only has the quality of instruction improved but new courses and curricula have been developed and implemented.

Inspectors in this period continued the on-going and intensive inspectional service in the field, at times making comprehensive surveys, at others dealing in depth with an aspect of the curriculum. Emphasis was placed on such curricular topics as: concurrent theory and practice, reduction of the heavy load of studies in the first year of the course, greater flexibility in methods of clinical teaching with provision for student participation, and the inclusion of experience and observational visits in psychiatric and public health nursing, respectively. In addition to preparing for and writing reports of visits, inspectors in the central office planned regional conferences and participated in committees of the professional association. Each inspector carried out a study related to the field, for example, the use of psychological tests and the role of the educational director in a school of nursing.

A development in nursing education which was to preclude a too narrow and literal interpretation of regulations was one in which the purpose and intent of legislation was adhered to as a guiding principle. A type of inspection service was planned to enable a greater number of persons in the schools and hospitals to participate in the evaluation of their particular programmes. This type of "self-evaluation" based on the objectives of the school was possible for a number of reasons: a democratic approach to supervision had been infused into the inspectional service since the beginning; the schools were receptive to the new idea; newer methods of working with groups of people on a co-operative basis were being used in the field of education. The result of this innovation was that each staff in resolving many of its problems moved toward its objectives at its own pace. This type of inspectional service was carried out by each inspector, or a team of inspectors, throughout the province. This new approach proved to be a strategic move on the part of the Nursing Branch, for it tended to reduce the possibility of excessive use of external and rigid controls. Actual experience in self-evaluation at home-base set the climate for, and was the forerunner of, the sophisticated conferences in which the profession participates today.

In keeping with the purpose and intent of legislation, the inspector assumed the role of consultant, although she retained the colloquial title, inspector, since its meaning was generally accepted. A consultant's role was possible, for, in most instances, the schools had moved far beyond the minimum standards. In making the decision whether to press for new minimum regulations or to promote the optimal objectives of the schools, it seemed that more was to be gained by the latter approach.

The balance achieved in this phase of growth gave each school the freedom to experiment and innovate within the existing legal framework. An example of the counterbalance to flexibility was the legislation enacted for the first time to regulate or control students' practice in the clinical field.[41] Both of these achievements had great significance for the future of nursing in Ontario.

In 1951, the Registered Nurses' Association of Ontario was authorized to administer the Act of that year. The inspection of schools of nursing, which for the most part were in public general hospitals coming within the Public Hospitals Act, 1931, was a statutory responsibility, which government did not delegate. Although the system of registration for registered nurses and certified nursing assistants was divided between two offices, the staff of the Association and the Nursing Branch worked closely, mainly through committees, to further nursing in Ontario.

In 1959, the Registered Nurses' Association of Ontario sought additional statutory powers to administer a practice act, and to supervise schools of nursing. However, the Association was advised that it was doubtful that statutory power would be given to an organization that did not represent all nurses, and, furthermore, that compulsory membership to represent all nurses would not receive favourable consideration.

A basis for government's decision as to whether a profession requires legal status and how it should be administered relates to the amount of responsibility that a profession carries.[42] Because of the "vital service"[43] that the individual nurse offers in her daily work, government deemed it necessary, in 1922, to establish a register to identify, for the public, nurses who were "qualified." Government in 1959, extended to the profession the privilege of considering increased autonomy. The suggested means by which this could be done was through the establishment of a statutory body, a College of Nurses.

The Registered Nurses' Association of Ontario recognized two principles in the idea of a self-governing body such as the proposed college: the right of the profession to determine standards of education and practice; and an elected body of nurses to administer the Act. The acceptance of these principles enabled the profession to establish the College of Nurses of Ontario[44] to administer the Nurses' Act, 1961–62.

The delegation of authority to the College is an acknowledgment that the profession knows, better than any other group of persons, what standards are required, and how best they can be implemented. On the other hand, the profession is mindful of its responsibility to

the people in proposing sound regulations to the Lieutenant Governor-in-Council for approval and in implementing legislation wisely.
It is through this mutual trust that effective relationships are built.

The College of Nurses of Ontario began its work with the educational programmes in schools of nursing and centres for nursing Assistants in March 1964. At the time the Nurses' Act 1961–62 was
passed, schools of nursing[45] had a total enrolment of 7997 students,
of which 3138 were admitted in September 1962. Basic nursing programmes leading to registration were offered by three universities,
the Nightingale School of Nursing (Ontario Hospital Services Commission), and fifty-eight hospitals. In addition, courses of approximately three months were available to most of the basic students in
the province in thirteen psychiatric hospitals, seven sanatoria, and
The Hospital for Sick Children. At this time more than 40,000
nurses were registered in Ontario.

AFTER 1970?

A newly created statutory body such as the College of Nurses of
Ontario, must, in a period of change, re-examine the prime purpose
it serves – the protection of the public. This principle was reiterated
in the recent report of the Royal Commission Inquiry into Civil
Rights after it had studied the statutes of twenty-two professions in
Ontario; "The granting of self-government is a delegation of legislative and judicial functions, and can only be justified as a safeguard
to public interest. The power is not conferred to give or reinforce
professional or occupational status. The relevant question is not 'do
the practitioners of this occupation desire the powers of self-government?' but 'is self-government necessary for the public?' "[46]

A registration authority, in studying how its members can competently serve the public, must examine the practice field to obtain a
reflection of the public's expectation of the profession. The need to
elevate nursing standards is important today, as it was at the turn of
the century, and what can be achieved in improving the quality of
nursing depends largely upon the kind of care that people want.
What nursing is to become will be determined by the public as it was
in 1872–96 when the service given by nurses trained under an apprenticeship system was both acceptable and economical, but without known standards or an educational base.

The statutes of all the associations in the health field in Ontario are presently being studied by the Committee on the Healing Arts, from the standpoint of the contribution that each makes to the service field. The report of the committee will be useful to the College of Nurses of Ontario in developing much needed legislation to regulate nursing practice. As well, the work of the Committee on the Healing Arts should bring about greater co-ordination between the health occupations and permit greater flexibility in interpreting regulations.

Although the functions of a registration authority may be many, its ultimate purpose remains the admission of applicants to the profession. This is the work of the College. How the College of Nurses of Ontario carries out its function depends to a great extent on the understanding that those responsible for implementation of legislation have as to the meaning and processes of law. Miss Fidler,[47] when the Registered Nurses' Association of Ontario was seeking control of the practice of nursing in the 1940s,[48] wrote: "It has become necessary that nurses should not only be familiar with the existing laws, but they should know something of the legislative machinery and approach to governmental bodies."

However, more is required than a background of the purpose and technicalities of nursing legislation. Each nurse in a position of responsibility must examine in broad terms her ideas about how the public can be protected from the indiscriminate practitioner; what the essentials of good nursing care are; and how educational principles can be transferred to the curricula of schools of nursing.

The understanding and knowledge that is essential cannot be left to chance. Programmes of study embracing law and the profession must be deliberately planned and carried out in a systematic and dynamic fashion through prescribed courses, conferences, and interdisciplinary seminars.

Control of the admission of "qualified" applicants bears scrutiny in times of change. In an age of specialization, uniformity of standards and centralization of control seems a less significant goal than it was fifty years ago. A registration authority today must study the type of recognition that should be given to registered nurses who have a high degree of skill, advanced theoretical preparation, and excellent clinical experience. If certification, the issuing of certificates in addition to registration, is to benefit the patient, ultimate questions which need to be studied relate to the powers of the controlling authority, categories of nurses to be provided for, admission requirements for courses of instruction, and types or grades of certificates to be given. If certification is not advisable one might ask whether a supplementary register should be maintained by the College of Nurses of Ontario for those registering beyond the basic level of competency. In this case a qualifying statement of the registrants' special qualifications might appear on the annual renewal certificates of registration.

In the problem of certification one must enquire whether the grouping of nurses into occupational specialties will tend to fragment the profession, or, on the other hand, if the Registered Nurses' Association of Ontario certifies these specialists, will the function of the College of Nurses of Ontario be restricted to the maintenance of minimum standards only? And, if this is so, is it desirable?

A prerequisite to admission to the profession is the provincial registration examinations. Whether there should be a multiportal system of admission to registration[49] should be explored, such as the exemption of approved schools of nursing with excellent standing from examination. Specifically, one might ask if graduates of the basic degree course in university schools of nursing could register without examination.

The control of the educational programmes and admission to schools of nursing is the means by which the registration authority can exert its greatest influence. The College of Nurses of Ontario in providing a consultative service, primarily to promote innovation, has answered a question which requires further study. The question is: What is the educational function of a registration authority?

As the staffs of schools of nursing become more proficient, what type of consultant service will be needed, and by whom will this educational decision be made? Are there other ways of fulfilling educational functions than by inspection or consultation, such as provision of a centre for information, statistical data, research, and consultation in special areas? Could a registration authority work on a co-operative basis with educational bodies in the evaluation of schools of nursing? If so, how could it be done?

A question correlated with educational function is that of goals. What will be the common characteristics of schools of nursing early in the next century? Should a registration authority provide leadership in the attainment of the profession's educational objectives? If so, how will it be done?

Answers to these and other questions will determine for the

College of Nurses of Ontario the nature and capacity of its growth. What will its official relationship be to the health professions and occupations, employers, schools of nursing, agencies, organizations and governmental bodies? How will it protect the public from the incompetent nurse? What is the responsibility of the College of Nurses of Ontario to be, in the rehabilitation of certain persons whose conduct has been such that it requires disciplinary action?

As the College of Nurses of Ontario re-examines its prime purpose and implements new legislation, it must of necessity study the events surrounding, and the meaning of, early nursing legislation. Only then will its members, the profession, see the foundation from which nursing in Ontario has developed and understand that "at once the law serves with its legacy from the past and with formulae flexible enough to hold the values of the future. Like the culture it serves, the law preserves its continuity with a constant change in identity".[50]

NOTES

1 Richard B. Splane, *Social Welfare in Ontario: 1791-1893: A Study of Public Welfare Administration* (Toronto, 1965), p. 196.
2 *Ibid.,* pp. 59-60.
3 *Ibid.,* pp. 46-53.
4 Ontario Department of Health, Hospitals Division, *Hospitals of Ontario: A Short History* (Toronto, 1934), p. 18.
5 *Ontario Sessional Papers, 1879*, vol. XI, no. 8, part III, pp. 1-3.
6 *Ibid.,* p. 212.
7 *Ibid., 1884*, vol. XVI, no. 16, part VI, p. 2.
8 *Ibid., 1883*, vol. XV, no. 8, part IV, p. 39.
9 *Ibid., 1879*, vol. XI, no. 8, part III, p. 21.
10 Sir William Osler, "Editors Miscellany," *American Journal of Nursing* V (May 1905): 529.
11 Isabel Hampton Robb, "Address of President" read before the Third Annual Convention of the Associated Alumnae of Trained Nurses in United States held in New York, May 1900. *American Journal of Nursing,* I (November 1900): 101.
12 Mary Agnes Snively, "The Toronto General Hospital Training School for Nurses," *Canadian Nurse* I (March 1905): 9.
13 Mary M. Roberts, "Modern Nursing 1873-1948," *American Journal of Nursing* XLVIII (May 1948): 277.
14 Sophie Palmer, "Training School Alumnae Associations," *First and*

Second Annual Report of the American Society of Superintendents of Training Schools for Nurses (Harrisburg, Pa., 1897), p. 55.

15 Graduate Nurses' Association of Ontario. Constitution and By-Laws (Toronto, 1910), Article II, p. 1.

16 Cecil Woodham-Smith, *Florence Nightingale 1820–1910* (London, 1950), p. 594.

17 *Ibid.*, p. 570.

18 Brien Abel-Smith, *A History of the Nursing Profession* (London, 1950), p. 242.

19 Rosa Shaw, *Proud Heritage: A History of the National Council of Women of Canada* (Toronto, 1957), p. 40.

20 Mary Ard MacKenzie, "Registration for Nurses," *Canadian Nurse* x (1914): 503–4.

21 Editorial comment, "Progress in State Registration in Canada," *American Journal of Nursing* VI (April 1906): 422–4.

22 Newspaper Hansard (microfilm). "Nurses Bill Has Been Held Over," Ontario Archives (20 April 1906).

23 *Ibid.*

24 *Ibid.*

25 *Medical Education in the United States and Canada.* A Report to the Carnegie Foundation for the Advancement of Teaching (Boston, 1910).

26 Royal Commission on Health Services, "Perspectives in Medical Education," in J. A. Macfarlane et al., *Medical Education in Canada* (Ottawa, 1965), p. 19.

27 *Royal Commission on Medical Education in Ontario.* "Supporting Statement H: Nurses," The Hon. Mr. Justice Hodgins, Commissioner, 1917 (Toronto, 1918), p. 162.

28 *Ibid.*, p. 43.

29 Ontario, Hospitals and Charitable Institutions Act, 1912, chap. 82, clause 18.

30 New York State, Nurse Practice Act, 1903, chaps. 203–9.

31 Registered Nurses' Association of Ontario, *Summary of History of the Graduate Nurses' Association of Ontario, 1904–1925*, presented at the First Annual Meeting of the Registered Nurses' Association of Ontario, Belleville, Ontario, 8 April 1926.

32 *Ontario Gazette*, Letters Patent: Registered Nurses' Association of Ontario, 4 December 1925.

33 Alexander M. Carr-Saunders and P. A. Wilson, *The Professions* (Oxford, 1933), part III, p. 351.

34 Ontario Department of Health, Nursing Branch, *An Analysis of Hospital Experience for Student Nurses in Schools of Nursing in Ontario* (Toronto, 1956).

35 Ontario, Nursing Act 1951, Regulation 455, clauses 21–4.

36 Ontario, *Minimum Curriculum for Approved Training Schools for Nurses in the Province of Ontario*, authorized by the Minister of Health, 1925.

37 "Education in Nursing, Provision of Nursing Care," *Report of the Ontario Health Survey Committee*, vol. 2 (October 1952), p. 277.

38 *Ibid.*

39 Canadian Nurses' Association, *A Proposed Curriculum for Schools of Nursing in Canada: A Tentative Report of the Curriculum Committee of the Nursing Education Section* (Montreal, 1936).

40 Ontario, Department of Health, *Curriculum and Information for Schools of Nursing in Ontario* (Toronto, 1948).

41 Ontario, Nursing Act 1951, Regulation 455, clauses 21–4. Amendment to the Nursing Act 1961–62, chap. 90, sec. 14(1), repealed.
42 Carr-Saunders and Wilson, *The Professions*, pp. 362–3.
43 *Ibid.*, p. 306.
44 Registered Nurses Association, "The Long Journey, Nursing Legislation," *News Bulletin* xvi (1960): 2, 3.
45 Ontario Department of Health, *Thirty-Eighth Annual Report for 1962*. "Nursing Branch," pp. 85, 86.
46 Ontario, *Royal Commission Inquiry into Civil Rights*, "The Power of Self Government" (Toronto, 1967), Report no. 1, vol. iii, chap. 79, p. 1162.
47 Nettie D. Fidler and Kenneth G. Gray, *Law and the Practice of Nursing* (Toronto, 1947), p. 102.
48 Registered Nurses' Association of Ontario, "Nurse Practice Act." References in connection with the Association's effort to obtain compulsory licensing and membership; and the resulting legislation which became law 30 March 1951 – Nurses' Registration Act 1951. "News Bulletin Excerpts" (Nov. 1945–March 1953).
49 Carr-Saunders and Wilson, *The Professions*, pp. 391–2.
50 Walton Hamilton, "The Law, the Economy and Moral Values" in Ward, A. D., ed., *Goals of Economic Life*, New York, 1953), p. 249.

3
Nursing as a profession

DOROTHY J. KERGIN

Almost two decades ago, Kathleen Russell pointed out that the nursing situation of the day "with all its confused struggles"[1] was the result of a trio of influences that began in the second half of the nineteenth century. The first of these she identified as the extraordinary developments in the practice of curative and preventive medicine; the second, the developing status of women and the new provisions for their education; and the third, a growing sense of social responsibility which focused attention upon the social and economic aspects of illness and health.[2] Today's concerns with the delivery of health services and universal medical care programmes, the socio-psychological aspects of illness, and the status of women in Canadian society are but extensions of these earlier influences that continue to affect the practice of nursing and the status of the nursing profession. Through the past century, nursing has evolved from a domestic service, characterized by Mrs. Gamp and her cohorts, to its present position as nearly a full-fledged profession.

Professional status and the concept of professionalism have been of increasing concern to nurses during recent decades. Davis, in his preface to five sociological essays on nursing, mentions the several paradoxes that characterize nursing. Among them he cites the fact that, whereas other occupations in America that are accorded the prestigious title of profession have established a baccalaureate degree as the minimum prerequisite for practice, nursing continues to rely overwhelmingly on the services of people who have not received a university education. The picture is further confused by the paradox that the terms "nurse" and "nursing" are used in popular parlance to describe a wide variety of personnel, working in many settings, and carrying out diverse activities.[3] Even the professional nursing organizations have difficulty in developing operational definitions of "nurse" and "nursing" that can be widely understood and accepted by their own members and those of allied professions, as well as broadly and clearly interpreted to the public at large.

The professionalization of an occupation is a complex process and, as Hughes suggests, is inevitably accompanied by a movement to set up categories of truly professional and less than professional people.[4] He would find this well illustrated by the present efforts of the professional nurses' associations in both Canada and the United States to distinguish between the university-prepared, or professional, nurse, and the diploma-prepared, or technical, nurse. Whatever else the term "profession" may mean, it is a symbol of high rank among occupations. If one regards the vocations of society as distributed along a continuum, with the well-recognized and accepted professions at one end and the least skilled and least attractive occupations at the other, then nursing can be generally located among the professions, with some variability with respect to the exact location of groups within nursing. This, as Hughes suggests, implies a distinction between nurses who can be considered truly professional and those who are somewhat less than professional.

Some have questioned the designation of nursing as a profession. Among the first was Flexner who observed over fifty years ago that "the responsibility of the trained nurse is neither original nor final."[5] At the same time, he identified six often-quoted characteristics of a profession which have been reiterated by numerous writers since his discourse.[6] The primary characteristics associated with professions are generally three: (1) they are based in a body of knowledge, growing out of science and learning and usually acquired through a rigorous period of formal education; (2) the members function independently, rendering a service to society that only they can provide; and (3) they formally organize into associations of practitioners. The practitioners, and the associations that speak for them, give high priority to the altruistic intent of the profession to place the interests of society above the interests of their own group. In return for this service on society's behalf, they ask of society a mandate to control the terms for entry into the profession, to regulate the conditions for remaining within it, and to set standards to govern the manner in which the service is rendered. The discussion that follows will consider the present development of nursing as a profession from the perspectives of professional education, professional practice, and professional associations. Some of the illustrative findings will be drawn from the writers' study of the professionalization of registered nurses in Ontario with respect to nursing education and educational change.[7]

PROFESSIONAL EDUCATION

Perhaps the greatest change since the time of Flexner's statement has been in the depth and breadth of knowledge and skill required by the nurse in order that she may fulfil her responsibilities. Except by a few reactionary physicians and nurses, she is no longer regarded as an amplification of the physician's skilled care. By the mid-twentieth century, instead of serving as a handmaiden to the physician, the registered nurse in hospitals became a member of the institution's bureaucratic structure, a facilitator and co-ordinator of patient care, and a manipulator of the patient's environment. It is interesting to note that Kathleen Russell identified the need for university preparation primarily for three groups of nurses – "the executive staff for hospitals, the teaching staff for all nursing schools, and ... public health nurses."[8] Although she called for much thought in the way in which hospital nursing was operating, she did not apparently foresee that the same societal changes that she identified would lead to a need for university-prepared nurses who would be closely involved in the provision of nursing care for patients and their families; nurses who would use their heads to guide their hands and conversation as they provided patient care that required a sound understanding of human nature as well as superb technical skill; nurses who would be capable of organizing and directing the work of others in addition to planning their own work in such ways that they reserved for themselves those tasks that required the competences of a professional nurse.

Conceptual Foundations

Charles Russell suggests that those who have studied the matter are convinced that "professional instruction should stress broad principles, key ideas, and overarching generalizations rather than detailed facts or techniques."[9] In nursing, curriculum development has been focused on developing the student's learning experiences around common problems of nursing practice. One group of writers has applied this problem-centred approach to the curricula of basic degree, diploma, and associate degree programmes.[10] The aim of the educational programme is to develop in the neophyte the capacity to cope with new demands for nursing care, not merely the ability to perform many nursing techniques that may be out-dated quickly as scientific advances make them obsolete.

In both hospital and extra-hospital settings, nurses are primary health workers with whom people have contact for extended periods of time. In all settings, it is important that there are nurses who are able to exercise responsible decision-making in planning, carrying out, and evaluating patient-care activities. These nurses must have a sound knowledge of human behaviour during the various stages of life, fundamental understanding of the physical, biological, and behavioural sciences, and skills in health teaching and promoting change that require insight into human motivation. The aim of basic baccalaureate programmes is to prepare professional nurses to meet these criteria.

The necessity for an education that emphasizes the basic principles of the scientific foundations of nursing is not limited to baccalaureate preparation but is equally applicable to other programmes that lead to a license to practise, the chief difference being a matter of breadth. For example, the newly developing two-year basic nursing programmes in Canada are planned with specific objectives in view for knowledge and skill, leading to competence in carrying out common nursing procedures.[11] However, acceptance of educational change develops slowly, and support of traditional programmes, in which there is an inclination to emphasize repetitive skills, remains strong among nurses. As recently as 1968, in a probability sample of over 500 Ontario registered nurses, approximately three-quarters of respondents without academic degrees and over one-third of those with academic degrees favoured the continuance of three-year diploma programmes, either in the traditional form in which theory and practice are interspersed throughout the three years or as three-year programmes in which the final year is a service or internship year.[12]

The Canadian Nurses' Association has taken a position supporting the concept of a diploma programme, planned within the framework of two to three years, and both the national association and its

provincial affiliates have encouraged innovation in nursing education and have spoken out strongly against an apprenticeship type of
programme. Nevertheless, the need for change in basic nursing education appears to have gained little more than grudging acceptance
throughout the profession as a whole. Recognition of the need for
change and of the capabilities of graduates of new programmes will
be slow in Canada until the sociological bases and the expected out-
comes of new programmes have been widely and rationally discussed among groups that extend into the grass roots of the professional organizations and until larger numbers of graduates of
basic baccalaureate and two-year diploma programmes are practising in well-established nursing fields, especially in hospitals.

Breadth

The present and future demands that face the nurse as a professional
and as a citizen indicate that the education providing the foundation
for professional practice must be obtained in a degree-conferring
institution. This is not a new suggestion. In 1948, Brown recommended that the term "professional" be restricted to graduates of
schools furnishing professional education "as that term has come to
be understood by educators."[13] This belief has been restated by the
Canadian Nurses' Association.[14] Yet the notion that it is desirable
to obtain basic nursing education through a university programme
has received limited endorsement and university programmes are
making a small, although increasingly larger, contribution toward
the preparation of nursing practitioners.* Among nurses registered
in Ontario, it appears that a majority of those without university
preparation and almost 18 per cent of those with university preparation consider new graduates of basic baccalaureate programmes
to be of little use at the bedside of patients, a primary practice setting
for nurses.[15] Whether this is due to an "anti-intellectualism" among
nurses, a phenomenon suggested by Reinkemeyer,[16] or whether it is
merely evidence of resistance to change can only be conjectured. In
the Ontario study, a majority of the respondents indicated that they

* In 1967, 273 nurses graduated from basic baccalaureate programmes,
compared to 7249 graduations from basic diploma programmes, or a ratio
of 1:27. For 1963, the reported ratio is 1:40. See, Table 9: "Ratio of
Graduations from Basic Baccalaureate Programmes to Graduations from
Initial Diploma Programmes of Professional Nursing in Canada, 1963–
1967," *Countdown 1968: Canadian Nursing Statistics* (Ottawa, 1968)
p. 72.

would encourage a new recruit to the profession to enrol in a university programme. A few justified their recommendation of the basic degree programme on the basis that university preparation was demanded by society. These nurses appeared to view it as necessary for promotional opportunities rather than for optimal patient care.[17] In the future, the position of nursing with respect to other professions will be greatly influenced by the extent to which nurses accept the principle that professional practice requires a broad educational preparation obtainable only in a university. It will also be determined by the proportion of its members who have attained at least this level of education.

Growth

The accumulating body of fact and theory in any professional field means that one can neither become nor remain expert without expanding, refreshing, and refining one's fund of knowledge and skill. Among the attributes of the professional listed by McGlothlin in his discussion of the aims of professional education are "zest for continued study which will steadily increase knowledge and skill needed for practice," and "competence in conducting and interpreting research so that he can add to human knowledge either through discovery or application of truths."[18]

This zest and competence must be stimulated during the undergraduate years and can be fuelled (or extinguished) by formal and informal educational experiences prompted by professional associations, employing agencies, and colleagues in nursing and related fields. However, zest and competence are maintained, not through external promotion, but by an individual dedication to the pursuit of excellence in nursing practice. As Henderson so clearly argues, "the nurse who operates under a definition that specifies an area of independent practice, or an area of expertness, *must* assume responsibility for identifying problems, for continually validating her function, for improving the methods she uses, and for measuring the effect of nursing care,"[19] and, "no profession, occupation, or industry in this age can evaluate adequately or improve its practice without research."[20] Responsibility for the enrichment of personal knowledge and skill and the expansion of the scientific and humanistic foundations of nursing practice must be accepted by nurses if they are to be considered professional and if nursing is to be regarded as

a profession. Yet, when one examines the Canadian nursing literature, the evidences of scholarly activity and creativity in nursing
practice are few. Most nurses will affirm that research and the application of research findings are important in nursing, but when a
sample of nurses was presented with a situation involving a new
nursing technique related to the care of a patient with a colostomy,
less than half suggested that the procedure be evaluated systemati-
cally. Indeed, the notion of carrying out a systematic study seemed
to occur to only one-fourth of nurses who reported they held no
university degree.[21]

The lack of scholarly activity by nurses will continue to limit the
degree to which examination of the theoretical foundations and
basic assumptions underlying the practice of nursing is carried out.
Research projects require financial assistance, but creativity and
curiosity do not. Nurse educators and administrators need to ask
themselves if they are exemplifying a creative approach to nursing
and are encouraging this in the students and staff with whom they
work. Individual nurses must examine the techniques and routines
that they too often seem to carry out mechanically, or as if Florence
Nightingale had decreed they should remain unchanged throughout
time.*

PROFESSIONAL PRACTICE

Two characteristics that are usually attributed to an occupation
identified as a profession are that it requires a large degree of individual responsibility in order to carry out its tasks and that it attracts
individuals who recognize their chosen occupation as a life work.
These will be considered as part of a general topic of professional
practice.

Independent Responsibility

Lesnick and Anderson, through the use of case material, discuss the
legal responsibilities of the registered nurse. On the basis of a study
of judicial decisions, they identified seven areas of professional nursing activity and have done much to clarify the nature of the nurse's

---

* They thereby disregard reports of the remarkably creative approaches that
  she engaged in to solve the problems that faced her.

independent functions. While they recognize that part of nursing involves the execution of legal medical orders, they state "the overwhelming number of functions and the majority of areas of control involve obligations of performance independent of medical orders."[22] One of the traditions of the past has been the admonition that "nurses do not diagnose." Yet, every day, nurses in various types of employment do diagnose, that is, they make judgments based upon their astute observations and their specialized knowledge. A diagnosis is formulated by the nurse in industry who must decide whether to send an injured employee home, to his doctor, or back to work; by the nurse in the hospital who deliberates whether to execute a physician's order for a p.r.n. medication for pain or to institute nursing measures to relieve discomfort; and by the public health nurse who must decide whether she, the physician, or the social worker, or all three, can bring the greatest amount of expertise to a family and assist them in solving their health-related problems.

During her educational programme or later practice, not every nurse is awakened to a responsible commitment that includes a desire to achieve the best in nursing practice, to be personally accountable for the calibre of the service that she renders, and to strive toward full awareness of the needs and desires of the individuals placed within her care. Like other occupational groups, there is a difference among individual nurses in the extent to which each exemplifies the attributes of a professional. In a study by Meyer, for instance, it is reported that the preferred work orientation of basic baccalaureate degree students tended more toward a "people" orientation in patient care, whereas diploma students were more "task" oriented. These patient-oriented values were retained by the baccalaureate group two years after their graduation, whereas registered nurses enrolled in a post-basic baccalaureate programme held values that were closer to those of the diploma students in the initial phase of the study.[23] Kergin reports that respondents with no preparation beyond a hospital diploma had a lesser tendency to recognize in a situation the failure of a nurse to provide emotional support to a patient preoperatively than did respondents who had earned university degrees.[24] Whether or not every nurse assumes her full responsibilities, independent areas of operation are present in nursing and each nurse is faced with situations that require sound judgments regarding her actions and those of the workers within her span of influence. Validity of these judgments regarding her actions is contingent upon rational and intuitive problem-solving methods, which require highly developed intellectual abilities.

Professional Commitment

Flexner describes professional activities as being "so absorbing in interest, so rich in duties and responsibilities, that they completely engage their votaries."[25] Yet, the conventional notions of the professions grew up in a world of men. In commenting on the view that a professional person commits himself to his work for his lifetime, Hughes and his associates point out that women are frequently faced with the task of resolving the relationship between career and family responsibilities.[26] Especially during their early work years, professional women often look forward to a limited or interrupted occupational life. The anticipation of establishing a home and family may interfere with their involvement within a profession. Indeed, large numbers of nurses, being female, move in and out of employment as their family responsibilities permit and in accord with the demands of the marketplace. Full commitment in the sense that Flexner's statement implies may be deferred until later years and may be attained by only a few.

In summarizing the several studies sponsored by the American Nurses' Association, Hughes and his colleagues cite the number of nurses who reported that they would remain in nursing, if they worked at all, as evidence of professional dedication and devotion "after the manner of women."[27] The majority of nurses in at least one Canadian province also appear to be relatively well satisfied with their career choices, since approximately 70 per cent indicated satisfaction with their selection of nursing as a career.[28] To the extent that satisfaction is an indication of career commitment, Ontario nurses, and probably most Canadian nurses, can generally be considered to be committed to nursing.

If commitment is measured by length of continuous service, then only a small proportion of nurses can be described in this way. Anderson, reporting for the United States, estimates that a third of women who enter nursing leave before completing their basic education and another third become inactive for long periods following a few years of service. The result is a small group of highly committed nurses who primarily occupy administrative and teaching positions.

"This is an unfavorable base on which to build a strong professional group because it would seem that any profession would need a high proportion of professionals from which to recruit for leadership, training and high level practice positions. The current educational and practice structure of the registered nurse is anything but encouraging to this type of professionalism."[29] His comments can be applied equally well to the Canadian nursing scene.

When considering commitment, one should not under-estimate the importance of the basic educational programme within which the individual begins to develop professional norms and values. It is during this period that the inculcation of these begins. If they are to develop a strong professional affiliation, recruits should be exposed to a professional and educational philosophy that will awaken them to professional responsibility and participation. Even so, upon graduation they may give higher primacy to goals of marriage and family life rather than occupational involvement, as the findings of at least one study suggest.[30]

Further insight into the problem of commitment in relation to nursing is provided in a study by Rossi. As nursing is changing it requires, more than ever, people who can be innovators and creators of knowledge or of new applications to nursing of knowledge gained in other fields. Rossi suggests that women of this type are more likely to be attracted to the traditionally male-dominated fields. She describes them as the "pioneers," women who are free of the need to be dependent on or nurturant of others; prepared to establish more egalitarian relationships with men, with people who are older than themselves, and with those in authority; and who are more likely to assume a stance regarding the roles of men and women that places them in positions of equal responsibility. These women have a greater willingness to participate in the job world, despite responsibilities of home management.[31] Robson, in his study on recruitment into nursing, reports that, compared to those who selected diploma programmes, girls who chose the university route into nursing were more concerned with having a job that involved interesting work, but were less likely to see nursing as satisfying them in this respect than were students in hospital schools.[32] It is quite possible that a number of Rossi's "pioneers," that is, creative and independent young women, now enter the nursing programmes of Canadian universities. As the more male-dominated fields become accessible to women, these young women who feel free to deviate from society's prescribed female role may be drawn into other occupations where they consider they have greater opportunities for personal fulfilment. This suggests that the nursing profession needs to examine, in particular, the image that it projects with respect to the university-prepared graduate, the nature of the responsibilities she can assume, and the potential opportunities for interesting and fulfilling positions awaiting her, many of them requiring graduate study.

PROFESSIONAL ASSOCIATIONS

Groups as large and complex as the professions require some kind of orderly procedure to set standards for entry into and exclusion from the occupation, to promote high standards of practice, and to raise the social and economic status of the group. It is also necessary for public or governmental agencies to know the thinking of a profession on particular issues. The professional associations provide the machinery for carrying out these functions. Carr-Saunders and Wilson express the opinion that "a number of men, though they perform similar functions, do not make a profession if they remain in isolation. A profession can be stated to exist when there are bonds between the practitioners, and these bonds can take but one shape – that of formal association."[33] Self-organization is therefore an important characteristic of a profession. In Canada, the professional nurses' organizations consist of the Canadian Nurses' Association and its ten provincial affiliates. The purposes of these eleven organizations are essentially to serve the best interests of the nursing profession and the public with respect to nursing, and to promote measures that lead to maintenance and improvement of standards of nursing education and nursing service. These measures generally include activities concerned with economic standards of employment.

Membership

In order for representatives to be able to express the weight of collective professional opinion, the organization of practitioners must be as comprehensive as possible. Even with a large membership, there is a danger that the thinking of an active minority will be expressed rather than that of the inactive majority. The professional associations must achieve the delicate balance of speaking for the profession as a whole and yet provide for the expression of dissent, striving to achieve what Merton terms "a flexible consensus of values and policies."[84] A comprehensive membership is facilitated in all provinces except Ontario by virtue of the fact that nurses holding active or practising registration in the province are also members of the professional association. In Ontario, the province that accounts for about 40 per cent of the total number of registered nurses in Canada, licensure and membership are separate. While there were approximately 54,104 nurses registered and resident in the province in 1968, the Registered Nurses' Association of Ontario reported a membership of 12,269, indicating that many nurses do not aspire to professional association membership, particularly when such membership is not tied to a licensing requirement.*

The problems experienced within the professional associations of trying to achieve a consensus among members on matters of professional concern is very much a matter of establishing effective channels of communication. This is difficult to accomplish satisfactorily when the members are as dispersed as are Canadian nurses. It is promoted through the publishing of *The Canadian Nurse* by the national association, through periodic bulletins by the provincial affiliates, and by the issuing of occasional pamphlets, brochures, and reports dealing with official positions, standards of education and practice, or special studies. As well, annual or biennial general meetings are held. There are indications that these methods do not adequately serve the communication needs of the profession. For example, in the Ontario study, approximately 50 per cent of association members did not appear to know what the stated position of the Canadian Nurses' Association was with respect to basic nursing educational programmes. Members with academic degrees seemed to be more knowledgeable regarding the Association's statements than were non-members with academic degrees, but for those with little beyond a diploma in nursing, membership appeared to have no relation to knowledge – members and non-members were equally ill-informed.[85]

The lack of well-established channels of two-way communication may result in a deceptive image of harmony. Bucher and Strauss warn of the danger of a spurious unity due to the power of certain groups within a profession and suggest that those who control the

---

* This is not to say that the situation is any different in the other nine provinces, if one considers only the proportion of the membership that is active in association activities.

professional associations also control the organs of public relations so that the outsider is unaware of any power struggles or discord.[86] Those who have been appointed and elected as the profession's leaders may have to make decisions regarding matters that have not been widely discussed throughout the profession. When this is necessary it is important that the decisions and the rationale behind them be thoroughly explored and discussed within groups that extend into the membership. Publication of official statements in professional journals and other means of written communication appear to be inadequate methods of reaching a large proportion of the nursing profession. As one Canadian nursing educator has said, "difficult and perhaps costly, though its accomplishment may be, failure to achieve an understanding, articulate, and actively supportive membership may prove a serious stumbling block to the attainment of desired goals, particularly in the field of education."[37]

Rational but fervent discussions at the local chapter level should help to produce excitement and understanding concerning the prospects and promises of change as well as creating a source from which the opinions and beliefs of the rank-and-file members can be forwarded to the profession's leaders.

Professional Ethics

Among the principles cited by Marshall as forming the policy base of professional associations is the imposition of a code of ethics, "which includes the duty to offer service whenever and wherever it is required, to give the best, to abstain from competition, advertisement, and all commercial haggling, and to respect the confidence of clients."[38] Codes of ethics generally embody in their statements an altruistic ideal of service to society rather than to self or to professional group. The Canadian Nurses' Association has adopted as its code of ethics the ethical code of the International Council of Nurses which states specifically that "service to mankind is the primary function of nurses and the reason for the existence of the nursing profession."[39] Whether formally codified or not the ethical principles of service are part of the professional norms and values that are transmitted to the nurse by example and precept during her early professional years, thus becoming part of the standard by which she measures her own performance and that of her colleagues. What the ethic of service is for the profession as a whole, a sense of altruism is for the individual. For the first, the interests of society are placed above the interests of the profession, and for the second, the needs of the patient are placed before those of the individual nurse.

Collective Bargaining

Any discussion of professional ethics leads naturally into an area of concern that some consider to be in conflict with a profession's ethical principles, that of collective negotiations or collective bargaining. Troubling to a professional organization is the time when it must reconcile its ethic of service with its efforts to achieve favourable conditions of work for its members. These members frequently view the problem of conditions of employment from different work orientations, some as salaried non-management employees, others with the bias of management. Both groups listen best to arguments that support their own points of view. One nurse regards economic security for nurses as a means to an end, thus reconciling the aims of collective bargaining with the profession's service ideals. She cites the real issue at stake to be, not just better personnel policies, but the matter of who shall control nursing, nursing practice, and the quality of nursing care.[40] A well-known social scientist, speaking to nurses attending an international conference, expressed the opinion that "a profession implies that the quality of the work done by its members is of greater importance in their own eyes and in the eyes of society than the economic rewards they earn."[41] Unfortunately, matters of salary and personnel policies are the concrete and tangible issues that can be argued at the bargaining table. Disparities in economic returns as compared with those of other occupations are much easier to validate than are those conditions of work which preclude the provision of the highest quality of patient care.

The 1960s have seen the professional nurses' associations in Canada becoming increasingly committed to the principle of collective bargaining by nurses, an activity that threatens to splinter these same organizations. Data concerning the disparity in beliefs related to collective bargaining, as held by management and non-management nurses, appear in Table 1.* At the staff level, it appears that

* These are part of the previously unpublished data collected by Kergin at the time of the study involving a sample of Ontario Nurses. See Kergin, "Professionalization," pp. 108–15 for other data related to collective bargaining.

TABLE 1

Opinions Regarding the Most Important Issue Facing the Nursing Profession with Respect to Collective Bargaining, Related to Respondent's Employment Position

Most important issue	General-duty or staff nurse		Above staff*	
	No.	%	No.	%
The status of women as nurses or employees	9	4	9	3
The need to distinguish between professional and union negotiations	53	24	52	19
The improvement of salaries and personnel policies for individual nurses	101	46	94	34
The desirability for nurses to influence nursing practice	14	6	43	16
The provision of high quality patient care	45	20	75	28
TOTAL	222	100	273	100

$X^2 = 18.58$; $df = 4$; significant at the 0.001 level.
*Assistant head nurse and above, including instructor.

over 45 per cent of the staff nurses in the sample considered the major issue to be the improvement of salaries and personnel policies for individual nurses, whereas among those who were appointed above a first-level position, almost 45 per cent indicated that the primary issue was either the desirability for nurses to influence nursing practice or the provision of high-quality patient care. Although many nurses may consider that higher salaries will lead to improvements in patient care, this is but one means to a desirable end. These data provide support for the view that the professional associations need to develop standards other than those related to salaries if they are going to gain the wholehearted support of their membership in collective bargaining activities. They must specify by what criteria the performance of nursing personnel with different types of educational preparation can be judged and indicate what nurses with differing levels of education can legitimately expect from employers with respect to continuing educational programmes, sabbatical leaves for professional enrichment, and promotional opportunities for demonstrated clinical competence. Above all, they must provide guidelines for adequate staffing patterns to promote effective patient care. Under enlightened leadership, nurses can help to make collective bargaining by professionals a desirable and respectable means for using the power of group action to improve the quality of health services.

In a world that seems, on the one hand, to be torn by strife and unhappiness and, on the other, to be reaching toward the achievement of standards of living unparalleled during man's tenure on earth, in company with many other professions, nursing is in a stage of ferment and growth. No profession can consider that it may stand still, and this has been recognized by nursing. The progress and acceptance of educational change has been discussed, as has the necessity for continuous examination of nursing practice and the effect of the intervention of nurses upon the health status of those for whom they care. The role of the professional association as a mediator between society and its members, a spokesman on professional issues, and a social mechanism for protecting the public from unscrupulous practitioners and its own members from unreasonable demands, has been examined. It is apparent that the professional nurses' associations must be strengthened in order that they may make a greater impact upon the quality of patient care and more effectively exercise the collective responsibilities of the profession. Their true influence will be felt when effective channels of communication operate throughout the associations and the strength of a large membership can be mobilized to influence decisions that are of consequence to nursing.

What is the present stage of development of nursing as a profession? Nursing is as highly professionalized at it believes itself to be. Faith in its precepts and foundations, confidence in its ability to change and innovate, wisdom in its choice of leaders, and a continuous desire to serve society's health and illness needs – if united in these, then nursing need have no doubts about its professional status.

NOTES

1 E. Kathleen Russell, "A Half Century of Progress in Nursing," *New England Journal of Medicine* CCXLIV (22 March 1951): 439.
2 *Ibid.*

62   NURSING AS A PROFESSION

3 Fred Davis, ed., *The Nursing Profession* (New York, 1966), pp. vii-viii.
4 Everett C. Hughes, *Men and Their Work* (Glencoe, Ill., 1958), p. 135.
5 Abraham Flexner, "Is Social Work a Profession?" in *Proceedings of the National Conference of Charities and Correction* (Chicago, 1915), p. 582.
6 For instance, see Odin W. Anderson, *Toward an Unambiguous Profession? A Review of Nursing, Health Administration Perspectives Number A6* (Chicago, 1968), pp. 10–11; Howard S. Becker, "The Nature of a Profession," in *Education for the Professions: the 61st Yearbook of the National Society for the Study of Education,* ed. Nelson B. Henry (Chicago, 1962), pp. 35–8; and Ernest Greenwood, "Attributes of a Profession," *Social Work* II (July 1957): 44.
7 Dorothy J. Kergin, "An Exploratory Study of the Professionalization of Registered Nurses in Ontario and the Implications for the Support of Change in Basic Nursing Educational Programs" (unpublished Ph.D. dissertation, University of Michigan, 1968); hereafter cited as "Professionalization."
8 Russell, "A Half Century of Progress in Nursing," p. 444.
9 Charles H. Russell, *Liberal Education and Nursing* (New York, 1959), p. 15.
10 Faye G. Abdellah et al., *Patient-Centered Approaches to Nursing* (New York, 1960), pp. 69–181.
11 Margaret E. Steed, "Trends in Diploma Nursing Education," *Canadian Nurse* LXIV (February 1968): 40.
12 Kergin, "Professionalization," p. 93.
13 Esther Lucile Brown, *Nursing for the Future* (New York, 1948), p. 77.
14 Canadian Nurses' Association, *The Leaf and the Lamp* (Ottawa, 1968), p. 4.
15 Kergin, "Professionalization," Table 21, p. 129.
16 Sister Mary Hubert Reinkemeyer, "A Nursing Paradox," *Nursing Research* XVII (January-February 1968): 6–8.
17 Kergin, "Professionalization," p. 151.
18 William J. McGlothlin, *Patterns of Professional Education* (New York, 1960), p. 7.
19 Virginia Henderson, *The Nature of Nursing* (New York, 1966), p. 38.
20 *Ibid.,* p. 39.
21 Kergin, "Professionalization," Table 24, p. 138.
22 Milton J. Lesnik and Bernice E. Anderson, *Nursing Practice and the Law* (2nd ed., Philadelphia, 1955), p. 261.
23 Genevieve Rogge Meyer, *Tenderness and Technique: Nursing Values in Transition* (Los Angeles, 1960), p. 117.
24 Kergin, "Professionalization," p. 144.
25 Flexner, "Is Social Work a Profession?" p. 146.
26 Everett C. Hughes, Helen MacGill Hughes, and Irwin Deutscher, *Twenty Thousand Nurses Tell Their Story* (Philadelphia, 1958), p. 239.
27 *Ibid.*
28 Kergin, "Professionalization," p. 146.
29 Anderson, *Toward an Unambiguous Profession,* p. 11.
30 Fred Davis, Virginia L. Olesen, and Elvi Waik Whittaker, "Problems and Issues in Collegiate Nursing Education," in *The Nursing Profession,* ed. Fred Davis (New York, 1966), pp. 153–4.
31 Alice S. Rossi, "Barriers to the Career Choice of Engineering, Medicine, or Science among American Women," in *Women and the Scientific*

Professions, eds. Jacqueline A. Mattfield and Carol Van Aken (Cambridge, Mass., 1965), pp. 80–4.

32 Reginald A. H. Robson, *Sociological Factors Affecting Recruitment into the Nursing Profession: A Report prepared for the Royal Commission on Health Services* (Ottawa, 1967), p. 106.

33 Alexander M. Carr-Saunders and P. A. Wilson, *The Professions* (Oxford, 1933), p. 298.

34 Robert K. Merton, "The Functions of the Professional Association," *American Journal of Nursing* LVIII (January 1958): 53.

35 Kergin, "Professionalization," pp. 93–5.

36 Rue Bucher and Anselm Strauss, "Professions in Process," *American Journal of Sociology* LXVI (January 1961): 332.

37 Evelyn Mallory, "Whither Are We Tending ... Updated," Paper presented at the Executive Committee Meeting, Canadian Nurses' Association, Ottawa, February 1964, p. 21.

38 T. H. Marshall, "The Recent History of Professionalism in Relation to Social Structure and Social Policy," *Canadian Journal of Economics and Political Science* V (August 1939): 327.

39 International Council of Nurses, *Code of Ethics*, adopted by the ICN Grand Council in São Paulo, Brazil, July 1953 and revised by the ICN Grand Council, Frankfurt, Germany, June 1965 (available from the Canadian Nurses' Association, Ottawa).

40 Dorothy Kelly, "Professionals and Economic Security: The Situation in Nursing," *American Journal of Nursing* LXV (January 1965): 78.

41 Marie Jahoda, "Nursing as a Profession," *Canadian Nurse* LXVII (September 1961): 826. (Italics in original omitted here.)

PART TWO EDUCATION FOR THE PRACTICE OF
NURSING: 1920–1970

4
The development of university nursing education

M. KATHLEEN KING

Nursing education became established on Canadian university campuses between 1920 and 1970. Its growth particularly in the early years was diffuse, and this led to such a diverse offering of courses and preparations that, to describe it in one chapter, we must narrow our focus and concentrate on undergraduate and graduate nursing education.

At present in the undergraduate programmes two courses of study are offered – the basic and the post-diploma programmes. The basic baccalaureate programme is an initial preparation in nursing; it lasts over a four- or five-year period and qualifies the student for a bachelor's degree and also qualifies her to write registration (RN) examinations. The post-diploma programmes, of two or three years, are offered to nurses who have graduated from a diploma school of nursing and who have qualified to write registration examinations before entering university. In order to be eligible for graduate study the student must have successfully completed a baccalaureate course and be admissible to the graduate school.

The number of graduates from all of the programmes is small. In 1968, 300 students graduated from the basic degree courses and 16 nurses received master's degrees. In the same year 7591 nurses graduated from diploma programmes. Of the 7891 nurses graduating in Canada in 1968, approximately 3.8 per cent graduated from basic university programmes. In addition, 667 nurses graduated from post-diploma baccalaureate programmes.[1]

These figures and definitions out of context may be dull and meaningless, yet, placed in perspective, they may give rise to concern or rejoicing. In either situation they give a limited view of university nursing education at the present time. They do not and cannot begin to depict the effort or the problems involved in strengthening the educational base of this emerging profession. To understand their meaning it is necessary to examine the development of this segment of Canadian university nursing education with its attendant problems.

The years 1919 to 1921 are significant ones, for in that period the first degree programme was started at the University of British Columbia, and five other universities offered certificate courses to graduate nurses. These certificate courses, spread across the nation from Halifax to Vancouver, for the most part concentrated on a one-year preparation in public health nursing. This apparently sudden development was the result of work which started close to the beginning of the century.

In the late nineteenth and early part of the twentieth century, the nurse gave a very simple kind of bedside care, mostly custodial, with the attendant domestic activities consuming a large portion of her time. She was in no way equipped to share in the developments taking place either in medicine or in the new field of public health. The training of the nurse took place in hospitals, large and small, often highly specialized but all conducting schools of nursing to meet their own particular needs for nursing service. The nurse trainees were placed in the wards, seldom having time to be taught and frequently with no teacher to teach. Following a required period of time the hospital granted a diploma to the graduate. Anxiety was expressed across the country regarding the effect of such training on both the patient and the nurse. By the early nineteen hundreds there was indication of a marked decrease in the number of applicants for nurse training and concern for the standard of care was evident. Graduate nurses wanting further preparation for the roles they were required to assume in teaching and administration were seeking it in the United States and often did not return to Canada.

The first documentation concerning efforts to establish a university nursing programme in Canada appeared in 1905 when a memorandum was submitted by the Graduate Nurses' Association of Ontario to the University of Toronto requesting the university to "offer a course of training and education of nurses."[2] As the University was undergoing a major reorganization, the time was not considered propitious. In the same period, there is, unfortunately only passing reference made to conversations held with Queen's University, but these indicate that some thought was being given to nurses receiving a degree from that university.[3] The time, however, was not appropriate and further discussions and direct representations were discontinued.

Although no further direct request was made to a university, a small but dedicated and vocal nucleus of nurses recognized that to improve standards of practice and to obtain needed recognition, a different educational base was required. Three major trends highlighted the inadequacies of nurse training and served to further the argument for stronger preparation. Very briefly these focused on: the widening scope of medical practice, the awakening public concern regarding social welfare and health, and the probing examination of professional education.

In line with the general ferment in professional education evidenced in the early years of the century, a Special Committee on Nurse Education was convened by the Canadian National Association of Trained Nurses. The Committee included representation from two Canadian universities in the persons of President Falconer, University of Toronto, and Professor McLean, University of Manitoba. In the report of this committee in 1914 a number of remedies were suggested for existing problems, the major one being to "establish nurse training schools or colleges in connection with the educational system of each province." The Report recommended that regular basic courses be offered, and, in addition, special courses in "district and public health nursing, social service work, hospital administration, and in the training of teachers of nurses for which special certification will be given." The final recommendation of the Report is worthy of note: "that the whole matter be considered calmly – not from the personal standpoint, but from that of 'Summum Bonum'."[4] It was unfortunate that this Report should appear at a time when the thoughts and energies of Canadian nurses were directed toward a different goal – a total war effort.

The desire for and move toward improved educational standards was never entirely abandoned even during the war. In 1919 a survey was made of Canadian university presidents regarding their views on university nursing education.[5] The presidents of universities with limited facilities for the teaching of nursing expressed modest interest; those with the necessary resources were even less enthusiastic. The one exception was the president of the University of British Columbia who, possibly because of his previous experience at the University of Minnesota, was eager to start a university programme in nursing. A year later, in 1919, the first degree course in nursing was begun at the University of British Columbia.

This new course required two years of study at the university, two years in the hospital, followed by another year of study in the university. It was the Canadian prototype of the pattern which came to be known as the non-integrated course or the 2+2+1 course in which the university assumed no responsibility for the basic preparation in nursing. Such an approach was already firmly established for degree work in the United States and, although the decision to copy this pattern possibly was inevitable, it was a most unfortunate one, and it has served to confuse and hinder nursing education and nursing practice since its inception.

THE EARLY YEARS: 1920–40

Following the war of 1914–18, the Canadian Red Cross Society became increasingly aware of the need for improved health services within the country, and focused much of its effort and resources on the provision of more adequate nursing service, particularly in relation to the rapidly expanding field of public health nursing. The Society approached a number of universities to determine the feasibility of establishing nursing departments to assist in the preparation of the public health nurse. These discussions, combined with the offer of generous financial assistance to both the universities and the students, proved productive and resulted in the appearance of certificate courses at six universities* in 1920–21, with a total enrolment of 148 graduate nurses.[6]

These courses were welcomed both by nurses and employers of nurses. For the first time the initial preparation in nursing could be supplemented in Canada and possibly in the province in which the nurse lived. It was not long before the variety and number of courses increased until further preparation was available in public health

* Dalhousie University, University of Toronto, University of Western Ontario, University of British Columbia, University of Alberta. McGill University offered courses for public health nurses, teachers, and supervisors.

nursing, hospital clinical areas, and the teaching and administration of nursing.

In a number of universities these certificate courses became closely associated with the developing nursing degree programmes. Credit toward a nursing degree was given for certificate course work and as this practice continued the weaknesses became more apparent. Increasingly, it was accepted that certificate courses gave the graduate an area of specialization without recognizing that in most instances the graduate had neither the academic background nor the necessary time for the development of abilities required for specialization. Initially, certificate courses served a needed and useful function in that numbers of nurses could obtain further preparation in a one-year period. However, as medical care and health services increased in complexity these courses were unable to keep pace with the growing demands.

A closer examination of these early degree programmes highlights the wide variety of courses required in the university. Relatively little emphasis was placed on groupings or sequence of subjects; instead, attention was focused on a field of knowledge that might lend itself to direct application by the nurse and that would serve to shore up the initial nursing preparation. Just such a practical approach is indicated by a course description included in an article written in 1927, "to the lectures of the final year various departments of the University contribute – as they do in the first and second year – special courses being given by the Department of Education, Sociology, Geology, and Motor Mechanics to meet the needs of the nursing group."[7]

The most perplexing aspect of this 2+2+1 arrangement was its acceptance by the university. Students received their nursing preparation in a hospital school of nursing with the university having no authority over either the students or their course. The university conferred a degree for work over which it exercised no control. There were obvious difficulties for all concerned, but most immediately for the students. Two such sharply contrasting environments, one institution devoted solely to education, the other oriented mainly to service, made entirely different demands on the students. There was a discontinuity of studies not only in content but also in method and philosophy. This break in contact with the university had wide implications for both the student and the nursing profession. In the teaching of nursing great emphasis was placed on technical skill, following orders, and adhering to established practice; the intellectual component was subservient to the daily round.

These early non-integrated degree programmes, closely related as they were to hospital training and certificate courses, were a deterrent to the progress of nursing both in education and service. They produced confusion in the minds of nurses and others regarding the purpose of university nursing education and its relation to nursing practice. Nursing was not well served, as there was little attainment of new insights and needed objectivity. Students were least well served as they were encouraged to enter baccalaureate programmes in nursing that were second class in relation to other university programmes. In spite of these obvious weaknesses traditions die hard, particularly when bolstered by financial considerations.

THE MIDDLE YEARS: 1940–60

A period of just over twenty years elapsed before the introduction into the university of a new pattern of baccalaureate nursing preparation. This new plan, known as the integrated basic course, combined general education in the humanities and sciences with specialized education in nursing. The curriculum integrated the two aspects of professional education and was planned so that one would strengthen the other. The first such course was introduced at the University of Toronto in 1942.[8]

It is of particular interest that for the first time in a nursing undergraduate degree programme full authority and responsibility for the teaching of nursing rested in the university. The nursing courses were planned, taught, and evaluated by full-time university teaching staff. This simple fact, nonetheless, was a radical departure from existing degree programmes, the roots of which, by this time, had been firmly established in both Canada and the United States. The new integrated programme fundamentally changed university nursing education in Canada. It accepted an intellectual component in nursing and more clearly aligned the teaching of this emerging profession to that of the established professions within the university.

In the initial efforts to gain control of the teaching of nursing, the contact between the university schools and the hospitals was in relation to the specific requirements of the university students. Unlike medicine, the nursing school staff had no role in the direct provision of patient care. In the early stages of development there was wisdom in this division; however, over the years this pattern has outlived the original useful purpose and has become an unnecessary burden to both hospitals and university schools.

The interpretation of this new type of preparation for the most part was hesitant and uncertain. Initially there appeared to be both a desire and a need to prove that the graduate of such a programme was "as good as" a graduate from a traditional programme. That this was carried on over too long a period can be attributed to a variety of factors, three of which might be examined more closely: the public concept of the nurse, the ambivalent approach of nurses, and the university nursing school.

The erroneous public image of Florence Nightingale as the kindly, soothing, ministering angel of Scutari has been a double-edged sword for the nursing profession. Great public support was elicited for nursing, but the picture was so firmly implanted that in spite of tremendous medical developments and social changes, the nurse was still seen in her nineteenth-century role. Kathleen Russell wrote of this dilemma in her New Brunswick Study. "Undoubtedly, it is the assessment of nursing as merely a somewhat glamorized, but quite simple, form of bedside care that even now sways world-wide and community-wide opinion concerning the work itself and, consequently, concerning the preparation for this work, that is, the whole field of nursing education."[9] Why this concept of the nurse became so fixed is difficult to understand. In the first half of the century the preparation and the work of the nurse changed beyond all recognition. The basic education of the nurse covered a period lasting between two and six years in nursing schools. The work of the nurse had even greater variations: caring for the acutely ill, the chronically ill, the convalescent; in the hospital, the home, the factory; teaching students and patients; administering care to large numbers of people. Undoubtedly, there is a need to clarify and interpret the preparation and activity of the nurse. Until this clarification for nursing as a whole takes place, misunderstanding will exist regarding the difference in role and function of the nurse with a basic baccalaureate preparation.

Throughout the first part of the century, organized groups closely associated with health care, for one reason or another, appeared to favour maintaining the narrow custodial image of the nurse. This coupled with the apparent inability or unwillingness of nurses to interpret developments in both education and service, further strengthened the accepted image of the nurse.

The situation was all the more unfortunate when translated from public confusion to government bewilderment. Since university nursing education has always depended on funds channelled through the provincial governments, it is essential that the needs of nursing be interpreted clearly to this level of government.* It was inevitable that through the lack of clear interpretation of the need for and the role of the baccalaureate-prepared nurse, there would be financial difficulties for university degree programmes.

The question may well be asked why, if the general public was confused, were nurses content to accept this situation. Over the same period other professional groups successfully recognized the need for evolving new educational approaches and interpreting these changes to the public. Unfortunately, the mass of nurses was apathetic and lacked understanding of both the need for and the character of the change in basic nursing education controlled by the university.

Two recent studies have examined this division of nursing opinion. One[10] points out that disparity in educational preparation between groups of nurses brings into clear focus conflicts in nursing which affect nursing education. This difference becomes a critical factor both in the development of new educational programmes and in the outcome for the graduate of these programmes. The author makes this latter point clearly. "It is of little use proposing educational change at the national level, and attempting to legislate it at the provincial level, if the local environment forces the graduates prepared in new programmes to conform to role prescriptions that oppose the principles upon which their education has been based and that lead them to adapt to the pre-existing professional norms."[11]

A harsher interpretation of the same problem has been made in the second study. "Precisely what nurses did not want was the prime contribution the university could make to the profession, through students and graduates. Novel ideas, critical thought, innovative behaviour, independent judgment, were all regarded as inimical to

---

* Since 1920 university nursing schools have received generous financial support from the Canadian Red Cross Society and from American foundations. This support enabled schools to explore and develop nursing programmes which otherwise might not have been possible.

nursing ... By their very existence these programmes and their products implicitly questioned the perfection of the hospital training system and the traditionally trained nurse."[12]

What then of the university nursing schools? Surely this is where one would find the needed interpretation. Unfortunately, not even here is there clarity of purpose. University nursing programmes were handicapped by the lack of qualified staff. Until the commencement of the first integrated programme in 1942 nurses with degree preparation received their basic work in a hospital training course. This often resulted in university staff being recruited from graduates of the one-year certificate courses. The essence of nursing, however, continued to be taught, not by university staff, but by instructors in hospital schools. As late as 1940, of 211 instructors teaching in hospital training schools across Canada, 25 had a university degree, 142 had a diploma or certificate, and 44 had no preparation.[13] It was this group mainly who taught nursing to university students.

From the early history it is not surprising that there was a lack of qualified staff; in fact, a shortage might have been expected for the first few years following such a radical departure. The years passed, however, and the impetus was not sufficient for numbers of nurses to seek further preparation beyond the one-year certificate courses, which were generally accepted as adequate qualification. In part, this slow development may be accounted for by the low academic admission requirements to hospital training schools. Of the nurses who sought preparation beyond their initial training many had a long period of make-up before they were admissible to universities.

The difficulties for the nurse seeking advanced study were compounded by the fact that no graduate work in nursing was available in Canadian universities. Canadian nurses again looked to American universities, but this time for graduate degree preparation. The early graduate study, in many cases associated with schools of education, was highly specialized. All too frequently this resulted in a highly specialized graduate programme being superimposed on a technically oriental basic education. As Strauss writes: "Nurses did move into graduate education, within schools of education and in masters' programmes within schools of nursing, but remained quite outside the university nucleus of genuine graduate training."[14] "Since the nurses who attended schools of education were pragmatically oriented toward 'service', they found nothing particularly wrong with the educational fare offered them at those schools."[15]

The diversity of educational backgrounds found among the staff of university schools made it difficult for them to understand the university setting. This individual lack of basic understanding made for difficulty in the collective interpretation of the strengths of the new basic baccalaureate programmes.

During the late 1950s, however, there was increasing recognition of the strength of the integrated baccalaureate programmes. Although a number of university nursing divisions appreciated the value of this approach, there were many barriers to accepting such a change; hospitals were loath to relinquish control of student time and service, universities recognized the increased costs involved, and many nurses did not support such a move. Change, though slow, was in the air and by the end of the decade nearly half of the university schools were making efforts to offer courses comparable to other professional courses given in the university.

While undergraduate programmes were being developed and strengthened, there was no parallel development in graduate nursing education. Canadian nurses continued to go to graduate schools in the United States. This proved to be a very expensive preparation for the nurses and for the country, since many nurses on completion of their courses remained in the United States. There were advantages in that nurses returned with a variety of experience and preparation, and that the limited funds and resources available for university nursing education were channelled into strengthening the undergraduate programmes. The disadvantages, however, have become increasingly obvious over the years. The preparation of the practitioner assumed paramount importance, and little time was spent on the study of the practice or of the theory underlying the practice. This in turn delayed even further the development of graduate work in Canada. It was not until 1959 that the first master's course in nursing was offered at the University of Western Ontario.

In the first thirty years of university nursing programmes there was a tendency for each university group to act in isolation. Individual schools jealously guarded their autonomy and the differences between programmes hindered the effective establishment of any organization for mutual benefit. The result was that in the early stages of development there was no co-ordinated voice for university nursing. This lack of a united voice weakened the entire nursing profession at a period, in the late 'forties and 'fifties, when a new national philosophy toward health and welfare was emerging.

The fundamental changes being studied and discussed nationally indicated new trends and patterns in the provision of health services. To be a part of these developments professional medical workers had to face new challenges both in education and service. Although many nursing leaders over the years had studied and recommended changes in nursing education, they had not been successful in initiating the necessary action for change. Nursing service had been taken for granted and with increasing strain nursing education had managed to meet the existing demands for service. With indications of basic changes in the patterns of medical services it was obvious that time-worn patterns of nursing education would be inadequate to cope with the predicted needs of health care. The time had arrived to face honestly the problems of nursing education as they related to the giving of nursing service.

THE PRESENT: 1960–70

Nursing, by providing an established, stable, and comprehensive component in health care, was indispensable to the functioning of other health services. For this reason nursing became a concern not only of nurses but also of other groups planning for future health care. In 1961 the federal government established a Royal Commission on Health Services "to inquire into and report upon the existing facilities and the future need for health services for the people of Canada."[16] The establishment of the commission, coinciding as it did with a period when the winds of change were being felt by various nursing bodies and groups, served to focus thought and discussion on the future of nursing and its contribution to health services. Briefs submitted to the commission indicated great unanimity in proposals for change in nursing education and these, embodied in the recommendations of the report, showed the direction for future patterns of education.

The assumption was made that two categories of nurses would be required; one to function in leadership roles, the other to function as technically skilled bedside nurses. Both of these groups would be educated in the post-secondary school system. The Report of the Royal Commission of Health Services designated one category as "The graduate of a four- or five-year integrated basic university programme or of a shorter programme for university graduates. It is estimated that about 25 per cent of positions for nurses require this type and range of preparation. These are the instructors, supervisors, administrators, and nurses in other leading positions."[17]

This proposal laid the basis for a series of recommendations related to university nursing education. These included the following: existing university schools should be expanded, new university schools should be established both for baccalaureate and master's programmes, and all university schools of nursing should develop integrated bachelor-degree programmes. In further recommendations the Report proposed that federal funds, professional training grants, and the health facilities development funds be made available to facilitate the proposed expansion.

The sixties ushered in a new era for university nursing education. It was a period of expansion. Nurses recognized the need for further preparation and society recognized the need for more and better-qualified nurses. Many of the university schools were suddenly faced with demands that taxed their resources to the utmost. This "quantitative problem" had far-reaching effects in Canadian universities. By the early sixties enrolment had doubled since the mid-fifties, and it would double again by the late sixties. From 1955 to 1960 university nursing enrolment increased, but the increase was less than that experienced in other university divisions. In the sixties, however, enrolment in degree work in nursing expanded rapidly. In terms of basic preparation this reflects the trend toward increased numbers of graduates from secondary schools entering university. While this trend toward university education contributed in part to the increase in numbers in post-diploma baccalaureate degree programmes the main thrust here is due to the wide publicity given to the report of the Royal Commission on Health Services among nurses and the implementation of certain of the recommendations. The increase in numbers (shown in Table I) is more meaningful when examined in terms of the changing patterns within the programmes.

The major change was in the increase in the number of basic integrated baccalaureate programmes. In 1963 there were sixteen basic programmes, eight integrated and eight non-integrated; by 1967 there were twenty-six, nineteen integrated and seven non-integrated. Since 1963 there has been a significant change in patterns of enrolment in the basic programmes. "In 1963 admission to non-integrated baccalaureate programmes exceeded admissions to integrated programmes by 22 per cent; in 1965, a reversal occurred; and in 1967, admissions to integrated programmes consti-

TABLE 1
Full-Time Enrolment in University Nursing Programmes 1961–67

	Programme			
	Baccalaureate			
Year	Basic	Post-basic	Master's	Diploma/Certificate
1961*	950	235	25†	879
1964‡	1410	724	22	959
1967‡	1956	1367	54	440

*Helen K. Mussallem, *Nursing Education in Canada, a study prepared for the Royal Commission on Health Services*, (Ottawa: Queen's Printer, 1964), p. 91, Table 69.
†This figure is from a personal communication with the University of Western Ontario and McGill University.
‡Countdown, *1968: Canadian Nursing Statistics*, p. 70, Table 4; p. 76, Table 2.

tuted 97 per cent of all admissions to baccalaureate programmes."[18] The strain placed on university schools cannot be attributed solely to the increased numbers but is to a considerable degree the result of the change in the pattern of the programmes. The integrated course, in which the university school is responsible for the total nursing content, has different requirements related to both staff and teaching facilities than does the non-integrated course, which allows the diploma school to shoulder the prime responsibility for the teaching of nursing.

Within the six-year period from 1961 to 1967 the enrolment in the post-diploma baccalaureate courses increased nearly six times. During these years employing agencies began to require university preparation for various appointments. This coupled with recommendations of the nursing organizations, mirrored in the report of the Royal Commission on Health Services, that "two categories of nurses are required" led many diploma graduates to seek university preparation.

In recent years there has been some change in the pattern of post-diploma programmes. At present two types of programmes lead to the bachelor's degree; one continues to offer specialization in either a clinical or a functional area of nursing, the other offers no nursing specialization. The increasing number of generalized programmes reflects the belief that specialization in university education belongs at the graduate level.

Graduate work in nursing has developed slowly in Canada. In ten years the number of universities offering nursing on a graduate level has increased to four,* but the enrolment in these programmes continues to be small. Roughly, between one and two per cent of nurses enrolled in and graduating from degree courses are in graduate work. Several factors contribute to the slow progress of the existing graduate studies in nursing: the early courses concentrated on the functional areas of nursing at a time when there was increasing interest in furthering knowledge in the clinical aspects; the habit of looking to American universities or to other divisions of Canadian universities was firmly lodged; the greater variety of courses offered in the American universities as compared with Canadian universities; the lack of emphasis on graduate education in the established undergraduate programmes. Despite limited numbers there is evidence of interest in graduate preparation in Canada. A recent study of basic-course graduates of one university school of nursing revealed that, of the 255 nurses who had not obtained degrees beyond the baccalaureate level, 107 indicated that they would be interested in a graduate degree in nursing if such a degree were available at that university.[19]

These changes, all involving a greater emphasis on the teaching of nursing and many requiring a more selective use of clinical facilities combined with the expanded enrolment, have suddenly strained the resources of the university schools. The problem of maintaining quality in the face of quantity has assumed top priority for university nursing divisions. Two specific problems illustrate the situation; one, the acquisition of academic staff, and, two, the availability of clinical resources.

In 1967 fourteen nurses in Canada had doctoral degrees and nearly five hundred had master's degrees. These numbers do not begin to meet the demand for nurses with this preparation either by educational institutions or service agencies. This placed the nursing school, along with other professional schools in the university, in a highly competitive position for academic staff.

Parallel in time to the expansion of university nursing courses was the expansion of enrolment in diploma nursing schools. These schools undergoing major organizational and curricula changes, while facing considerable pressure to increase enrolment, required

* University of Western Ontario, McGill University, University of Montreal, University of British Columbia.

a variety of selected clinical settings in which to expand their programmes. The majority of diploma schools, still closely associated with hospitals, had priority of access to clinical facilities in the home hospital. This situation led to a limit being placed on enrolment by some of the university schools that could not obtain adequate clinical resources.

With the relatively recent achievement of sound basic baccalaureate programmes and of beginning graduate programmes, university nursing education is faced with the immediate challenge of change indicated by trends and new developments in the provision of health care. As the demands and needs for care increase, new approaches to the provision of health services are being studied, particularly as they relate to the effective use of the abilities of professional people. Before these changes can be adequately absorbed, university nursing schools need to focus their attention on three pressing problems: first, a clearer understanding of the abilities of basic baccalaureate graduates; second, a strengthening of relationships both in the university and in the clinical setting; and third, a greater emphasis on graduate programmes.

A clear understanding of the abilities of the basic baccalaureate graduate is essential if the talents and skills of the graduate are to be used effectively. The continuing demand for concise statements related to the specific capabilities of these graduates mirrors a lack of understanding of university education. That such a lack exists, may be attributed in part to the high degree of technical specialization associated with the early university nursing courses. The function of the university, however, is not to graduate head nurses, team leaders, staff nurses, or directors of nursing but rather, as Sidney Smith said, to "train for the higher ranks of the profession those with gifts for theory and talents for leadership and investigation."[20] A real effort has been made to relate the contribution made by the graduate to the existing structure of nursing and to fit her into the most appropriate place. The challenge is to interpret the abilities of the graduate in terms of the emerging patterns of health care. The onus for this explanation rests with the university nurse-educators.

The second need of the university nursing school is to review and strengthen relationships both in the university and in the clinical areas. Understanding is greatest when colleagues learn to appreciate the capabilities of one another on a co-operative basis. For university nursing staff and students these relationships cannot be carried on in isolation either in the university or in the clinical setting. The connection with the university is based on scholarship and scholarly activity, and as this tie is strengthened nursing will become more fully a part of the university. It behooves the schools to examine existing baccalaureate programmes to determine whether they do provide the necessary basis for graduate work, whether they are theoretical and liberal or whether, in fact, they are primarily practical and technical. Although such vigilance must be continuous, a more fundamental requirement is the involvement of teachers in research. Through the new insights gained, knowledge is extended and enthusiasm is transmitted to students who in turn seek new approaches.

Health science centres are evolving within many universities. This organization embracing all the health professions can provide unlimited opportunity for exploring problems of service and developing collaborative relationships among the professions. Throughout their education, students will be able to profit from the competencies of all members of the professional groups and this in turn will generate effective relationships. It can be expected that interdisciplinary research projects organized in these centres will make an increasing contribution to both health knowledge and health services. Nursing schools need to take the necessary measures to become integrally involved in this approach, where possible from the beginning and at least from the earliest opportunity.

In order to participate in these developments the university nursing school needs a closer association with the clinical settings – both institutions and community agencies. This need is twofold; first, nursing teachers should be and want to be involved in nursing practice, and, second, the school through its staff should be able to influence the standard of care in areas where students are taught. At the present time clinical fields are themselves facing new demands as patterns of care change. No longer can traditional methods of nursing care and forms of organization be accepted without question. New approaches based on sound theoretical knowledge, but flexible and easily adaptable to change, must be found to meet the demands.

To meet the challenge of promoting excellence in nursing practice, co-operation between education and service is a necessity. There is a pressing need to question, plan, and assess patterns of care as a basis for new approaches which will more readily adapt to growth and change. Nurses with sound knowledge and clinical expertise are needed to give leadership in these developments. In response to this need for clinically expert nurses who can give leadership in improving and establishing new patterns of patient care, graduate work in nursing must be expanded. The early programmes concentrated on the functional aspects of nursing, but, with an increasing need to expand knowledge of nursing specialties and to investigate improvements in nursing, new programmes are focusing on clinical specialization. These programmes are required both from the educational aspect of expanding knowledge and from the service aspect of increasing the nursing contribution to improved health care.

Graduate schools in the older Canadian universities developed as centres of scholarship in the purely theoretical subjects and, as such, recognized a responsibility to generate an expansion of knowledge in these disciplines. This underlying philosophy has affected admission to the graduate schools of professional faculties that are principally concerned with the application of knowledge derived from a combination of theoretical subjects. This has had not an altogether unsalutary effect on nursing. Although graduate work in nursing *per se* has been delayed, nurses have been forced to study and investigate their subject and from this effort a theoretical body of knowledge has emerged. Doubtless, this process would be more effectively pursued supported by the resources of the graduate schools. However, a degree or diploma is in itself valueless and becomes meaningful only as it represents an achievement of scholarship.

In recent years there has been a tendency to recognize the needs and the dilemma of the new professional schools. The indications of change within graduate schools combined with the work in nursing point the way to the early development of sound graduate programmes which will be directed toward clinical nursing specialties. An anniversary year, particularly a fiftieth anniversary year, bestows a licence to assess the development of nursing education within universities over the half century. On first glance the progress seems slow and lacking in vitality with no clear direction; however, two accomplishments in this period stand out clearly as strengths and good omens for the future – the introduction of the basic integrated baccalaureate degree programmes and the development of graduate work. These achievements are sound and the spirit of impatience engendered by the present must not unduly cloud the recognition that coming of age, like all processes of maturation, requires time. The lack of a university tradition has had a marked influence on the slow development of nursing within the universities. Nursing departments continued to have close and strong associations with professional nursing groups, and in the early phases of this relationship, the university schools were vulnerable to the fluctuating demands and pressures of these nursing groups. The schools for a period in their development found themselves in the unsatisfactory position of trying to be all things to all men. There has been a curious reluctance on the part of the university nursing schools to define clearly their role in the whole field of nursing education. Perhaps this might be attributed again to the early training and traditions of nursing when such words as "criticism" and "different" had strong negative emotional connotations.

The introduction of the basic integrated baccalaureate degree course was the key factor in relating nursing education to established forms of university professional preparation. This placed the responsibility for the teaching of nursing under the control of the university and as such placed the resources of the university behind the development of this new discipline. That nursing has been slow to utilize these resources should not, perhaps, have been unexpected. Through the years much nursing knowledge has been derived from the close experience of caring for people, sick and well, combined later with supporting knowledge derived from the sciences and humanities. Nursing staff, while being deeply involved in professional problems outside the university and in curriculum development within the university, could maintain considerable zest and enthusiasm in their teaching by the skilful use of clinical illustration. Unlike their university colleagues they did not possess the scholarly motivation for planned study and investigation of their subject.

The great social changes and the advances in the area of health care have changed the function and role of the nurse. These changes, combined with the increased number of nurses having graduate preparation, have served to focus attention on developing a body of nursing knowledge and on studying the practice of the profession. As one Canadian nurse-educator has written "it is clearly evident today that a scientific body of knowledge in nursing is emerging, that nursing can be theory rather than technique oriented and that it can be studied in a cause-effect relationship."[21] The development of this body of knowledge requiring study and investigation has changed both the content and method of teaching nursing in undergraduate programmes, but, of greater lasting importance, it has made possible the development of graduate education in nursing.

NOTES

1 Research Unit, Canadian Nurses' Association, 1969.
2 Agnes H. Paffard, "History of the Graduate Nurses' Association of Ontario," *Canadian Nurse* IX (May 1913): 298.
3 Society of Graduate Nurses of Ontario, "Minutes of the Second Annual Meeting," 22 April 1905.
4 Report of the Special Committee on Nurse Education, Fourth Annual Convention of the Canadian National Association of Trained Nurses, *Canadian Nurse* X (October 1914): 571–2.
5 Helen MacMurchy, "University Training for the Nursing Profession," *Canadian Nurse* XIV (September 1918): 1284–8.
6 Canadian Red Cross Society, "The Role of One Voluntary Organization in Canada's Health Services," A Brief presented to the Royal Commission on Health Services (May 1962), pp. 96–115.
7 Mabel F. Gray, II, "The Five Year Degree Course in Nursing in the University of British Columbia," *Nursing Education in Universities in Canada* (The International Council of Nurses, 1927), p. 189.
8 For further detail on this course at the University of Toronto see below Dr. H. M. Carpenter's article, "The University of Toronto School of Nursing, An Agent of Change."
9 Edith Kathleen Russell, *The Report of a Study of Nursing Education in New Brunswick* (Fredericton, 1956), pp. 21–2.
10 Dorothy J. Kergin, "An Exploratory Study of the Professionalization of Registered Nurses in Ontario and the Implication for the Support of Change in Basic Nursing Educational Programs," (unpublished Ph.D. dissertation, University of Michigan, 1968).
11 *Ibid.*, p. 169.
12 Sister Mary Herbert Reinkemeyer, "A Nursing Paradox," *Nursing Research* XVII (January-February 1968): 7.
13 Agnes J. MacLeod, "Nursing Education in Canada," *Canadian Nurse* XXXVI (October 1940): 666.
14 Anselm Strauss, "The Structure and Ideology of American Nursing," in *The Nursing Profession*, ed. Fred Davis (New York, 1966), p. 81.
15 *Ibid.*, p. 82.
16 Canada, *Royal Commission on Health Services Report*, vol. 1 "Greeting" (Ottawa, 1964).
17 *Ibid.*, p. 63.
18 *Countdown, 1968: Canadian Nursing Statistics* (Ottawa, 1968), p. 67.
19 Nora I. Parker, "Survey of Graduates of the University of Toronto Baccalaureate Course in Nursing" (Toronto, 1968), p. 38.
20 Sidney Smith, "President's Report for the Year Ended June 30, 1953–1954," pp. 17–18.
21 Alma E. Reid, "Report to the New Zealand University Grants Committee on Commonwealth Prestige Fellowship Assignment, 1965" (unpublished).

5
The University of Toronto School of Nursing: An agent of change

HELEN M. CARPENTER

The story of nursing education in the University of Toronto is essentially the story of Kathleen Russell's search for a better method of preparing nurses for their work. A graduate of King's College, Nova Scotia, and of the Toronto General Hospital School of Nursing, Kathleen Russell was appointed to direct the Department of Public Health Nursing in the University of Toronto when it was established in 1920. She remained in this post until her retirement in 1952, and throughout these years she strove to gain acceptance for the application of sound educational principles in schools of nursing. Her intellectual vigour, zeal, and fine personal qualities contributed to her success in selecting and holding a strong and dedicated staff who shared her aspirations and commitment to nursing. Together they introduced radical innovations in nursing education – innovations that have gained acceptance and have influenced the preparation of nurses in Canada and in many other countries.

Following the First World War, nurses were needed for service in the new field of public health. Trained as they were in the hospital schools, they were not prepared for this work. For several years, universities in the United States had offered specialized courses in public health nursing, but Canadians who enrolled were frequently lost to Canada. The Canadian Red Cross Society became interested in health education as a result of the diseases found among army recruits, and the recurrence of the influenza epidemic that swept the world following the war. With funds available after the cessation of hostilities, the Red Cross launched a programme to stimulate interest in health services and to disseminate knowledge concerning health through demonstration and education.[1] In 1920, the Ontario

Branch of the Society offered financial support to the university for an initial period of three years to establish a Department of Public Health Nursing. The offer was accepted and Kathleen Russell was appointed to direct the department. Preliminary work had been undertaken on the curriculum for a certificate course in public health nursing which was approved by the university Senate in May. The department was established in offices provided by the Faculty of Medicine with a staff consisting of the director and a supervisor of field work.*

1920: THE FIRST COURSE

The Public Health Nursing Course consisted of six months of theoretical work and three months of practice. Various departments contributed to the teaching, including those of hygiene, medicine, household science, and social service. Field work was arranged in co-operation with the Toronto Department of Public Health and other community agencies. A statement in one of the first calendars is indicative of the seriousness with which this work was viewed: "The student who approaches her field experience as a piece of individual research work will reap a greater benefit than the one who would enter merely as an apprentice to learn the technique of this work."[2]

From the outset, there was dissatisfaction with the course because of the lack of co-ordination between the students' basic training and preparation for public health nursing, and the department's lack of control over student selection.

... the public health nurse who has been prepared in this way for her work [wrote Kathleen Russell] has spent four years in the process of preparation, three years in the hospital, and one year in this special school. A close examination of the content of the four years shows that, from the standpoint of educational procedures, the whole arrangement is indefensible except upon the ground of emergency need. If we con-

* Associated with this development were: Colonel (Dr.) G. G. Nasmith; Miss Jean I. Gunn, Superintendent of Nurses, Toronto General Hospital; and Mrs. H. M. Plumptre of the Ontario Red Cross Society; the President of the University of Toronto, Sir Robert A. Falconer; Dr. J. G. Fitzgerald, Professor of Hygiene; and Dr. Duncan Graham of the Department of Medicine.

sider the product in relation to the time and energy expended ... this same product is sadly inadequate to meet the requirements of public health nursing and the result is most unfair to the student who has spent so much time upon an ill-arranged programme of studies.[3]

Admission was based on graduation from an "acceptable training school" and high-school education to grade eleven. Despite this control it was difficult to plan a satisfactory course. The curricula in the hospital schools were lacking in preliminary science work and relevant clinical experiences. In a one-year course it was difficult to alter the attitudes of students whose training had been confined to the care of the sick.

At this time the only avenue open to young women who wished to enter nursing was to enrol in a hospital school. In a report written in 1923 following a survey of the ninety Ontario schools, Edith MacPherson Dickson, the first inspector, wrote: "These training schools were not established with the idea of preparing young women to care for the sick, but rather as a means of providing an economical service to the sick in hospitals – a service which has always included a great deal of domestic work rather than purely nursing service."[4] No standards had been established for these schools. The level of education on admission varied widely, some students having public school education only. The service needs of the hospitals took precedence over the educational needs of the students. Graduate nursing staff was minimal or completely lacking. Theory and practice were unrelated. Clinical experiences needed by the students were not always available in the hospitals that established schools. In addition to nursing the patients, the students were required to undertake a variety of tasks needed for the smooth operation of the hospital, such as housekeeping, office routines, and management activities. Physicians accepted responsibility for teaching the students, but as they had busy practices, and in some instances also taught medical students, little time was available for planning and co-ordinating their lectures. Nursing instructors usually lacked special preparation, as no post-basic education was available in Ontario. Classroom and residence accommodation were sub-standard: "... the history of every hospital [wrote Miss Dickson] shows that provision of adequate hospital accommodation has always preceded the provision of even hygienic living conditions for those who must spend their entire day in the wards of the hospital."[5]

These conditions were a source of concern to nursing leaders. A similar situation in the United States led the Rockefeller Foundation to support a study of nursing education in that country.[6] Through its fellowship programme, the Foundation made possible the interchange of ideas between nursing leaders from a number of countries. Kathleen Russell was a recipient of a Rockefeller fellowship and the observations she made in the United States and England helped to shape her thoughts with regard to the reform of nursing education in Canada.

THE SEARCH FOR A BETTER WAY

A memorandum found among Miss Russell's papers reveals the first phase in her search for a new approach to nursing education. At this time she foresaw the need for nurses to be qualified for four types of work: bedside nursing of the sick, public health nursing, teaching, and administration. The possibility of providing three separate courses was considered with provision for later post-basic nursing education or university education in the Faculty of Arts. She thought a school of nursing should be affiliated with a university "to save duplication of work already provided there, [and] to find a path across to existing degree courses for the few able to follow such."[7] She considered two alternative plans: a new nursing school independent of but in close affiliation with the university and with the hospital wards and a public health nursing service at its disposal; or two institutions – a hospital nursing school specially staffed, and a nursing school in a university, or independent ... in close affiliation with the hospital.[8]

The desirability of relating the preventive and curative aspects of medicine in the education of doctors and nurses was recognized by Mary Beard of the Rockefeller Foundation.[9] Kathleen Russell shared this belief and in 1932 made a number of recommendations to guide the development of public health nursing education:

(1) that direct preparation of the public health nurse should be provided; the indirect method of adding a post-graduate year to the ordinary nurses' training is merely trifling with the matter;

(2) that a public health nurse should be trained to do bedside nursing;

(3) that the public health nurse must be prepared for state registration as a nurse;

(4) that this country is not ready to provide for registration of public health nurses as distinct from other nurses, and that, consequently, the public health nurses' training must include the minimum state requirements in bedside nursing;

(5) that the training in bedside nursing is necessarily of a somewhat prolonged nature; so that it will not be a sound proposition, from the economic standpoint, to add to the time spent in hospital a further great length of time to make up the total amount of the public health nursing training;

(6) that (consequent to 5) the time spent in hospital training should be utilized to the full as part of the training of the public health nurse;

(7) that (if we could pay our way) much could be done with the hospital training to make it contribute fully to the desired preparation of the public health nurse.

To lay a better foundation for public health nursing, changes in the training offered by hospital schools were recommended:

(1) that relevant hospital services be included: children's, communicable diseases, obstetrical, out-patients, tuberculosis, eye, ear, nose, and throat, mental, and social service;

(2) that some less-needed services be ruthlessly discarded;

(3) that hours of work be greatly reduced;

(4) that it be made possible for the so-called student to live the life of a student;

(5) that instructors with a knowledge of health work, and interest in it, surround the pupil throughout her hospital training.[10]

1926: THE FIRST EXPERIMENT

In an attempt to overcome the deficiencies of the certificate course, a diploma course was introduced in 1926. This four-year course consisted of two years in the university (the first and fourth years), and two years in a hospital school. A foundation was laid in the humanities and sciences in the first year, followed by two years in the School of Nursing of the Toronto General Hospital. The fourth year in the university completed the preparation in public health nursing. Graduates were awarded the diplomas of the Toronto General Hospital and of the university.

Although this course offered a better preparation than the certificate course, there were many undesirable features. It consisted of two unco-ordinated parts, each under a distinct authority. Despite the dissimilarity in their educational backgrounds, in the second and third years the university and hospital students were taught together by staff of the hospital school. Little co-ordination was possible between the content of the first year and that of the second and third years. The service requirements of the hospital militated against learning. The students were "on duty" over a twelve-hour period, seven days a week, with two half-days off. The twelve-hour day was broken by two hours "off duty" except on days in which classes were scheduled in this period. To graduate, the students were required to complete the fourth year and to "make up" any time they had lost through illness during the second and third years.

As one would expect, Kathleen Russell was far from satisfied with this course, and in looking back upon it after it had been discontinued, wrote: "We would never willingly return to that four-year course as it has been conducted; it was a gruelling experience for the students which only allowed for the survival of the fittest."[11]

THE STRUGGLE TO ESTABLISH THE SCHOOL

It took twenty-five years of painstaking study and planning to achieve a university degree course in nursing. A steady exchange of correspondence between Kathleen Russell and Mary Beard reflects the intensive work undertaken between 1926 and 1933 to establish the School of Nursing in the University of Toronto. The Department of Public Health Nursing moved to the School of Hygiene in 1927. With financial assistance provided by the Rockefeller Foundation the school was able to secure a new building for the expansion of its programme and an arrangement was made whereby the Department of Public Health Nursing was accepted as a sub-department in the School of Hygiene. This arrangement was a distinct advantage for the department as it provided an association with a strong programme of research and teaching in a school that had gained wide recognition and respect for its contribution to preventive medicine and public health.

In 1928 consideration was given to expanding the work of the department by developing a second certificate course to prepare graduate nurses for teaching and administration. Although the School of Hygiene supported Miss Russell's goals for nursing education, it appeared inappropriate to broaden the programme beyond that considered to be a proper function of the school. The course in teaching and administration was therefore established in the Division of Extension.

A plan for one unified School of Nursing to include the courses offered by the Department of Public Health Nursing and the Division of Extension was submitted to the Rockefeller Foundation in 1929. Although the foundation was favourably disposed toward this proposal, support was contingent upon the response of the university and the Ontario government. Correspondence with Mary Beard reflects the spirit in which Kathleen Russell launched upon negotiations:

... I think I may say that in our own peculiarly slow fashion we have really made satisfactory progress. But we are very slow! However, there is nothing else for me to do than to take things – and people – as they are and work with them in their own way. At last we have seen the Prime Minister, Mr. Ferguson, but only yesterday. Miss Gunn and I saw him together and in company with Sir Joseph Flavelle. And thereby hangs a very long tale. Sir Joseph is a member of the Board of Governors of the University and also of the Toronto General Hospital, and is a man of very great prestige in the business world. He has given us valuable help in presenting our case.

Of course the Prime Minister made no commitment of any kind yesterday but he did give a very satisfactory hearing to the matter. I think he is sincerely and intelligently interested in nursing. There was less of nonsense in this interview with him than in most where nursing is under discussion.

Meantime, a sympathetic understanding of our proposition has been growing among a few of our most influential friends and I am really amazed to see how acceptable the project has become. I think we have good reason to hope that it can be carried through successfully. How different was my feeling when I drew up those recommendations in September![12]

During this period Kathleen Russell was actively engaged in interpreting the proposal to colleagues in the medical and nursing professions and associates in the hospitals and other health agencies. She saw an intimate connection between nursing and medicine, stating that "the nursing school cannot be considered apart from the medical school and therefore, some degree of association must be arranged between the two."[13]

It was with a deep sense of accomplishment that she responded to the communication from the Faculty of Medicine, when in 1930 the Council of that Faculty approved in principle the proposal for a School of Nursing in the university. In a letter to the Dean of Medicine she wrote "We are only at the beginning of a lengthy process in shaping the details of these plans, but once we can be assured of a proper relationship with the Faculty of Medicine, the plans can be worked out safely and wisely; this will only be a matter of time."[14]

Meanwhile, negotiations with the government were delayed by the resignation of the Prime Minister in 1931, and Miss Russell was faced with the need to interpret the plan to a new Prime Minister and a new Minister of Health. As by this time the country was in the depths of an economic depression and there was unemployment among nurses, the proposal for a university school of nursing met with the objection that it would add one more school to a number already overly large. Kathleen Russell contended that the proposed school was to be associated with the Toronto General Hospital for clinical work, and in view of this, the new university school would provide "a re-arrangement of training in *connection with a group of pupils already in existence.*" She expressed concern about the "overproduction of nurses," and the "too high cost of nursing service ... for the average consumer," and pleaded for "an opportunity to work quietly and constructively toward a solution of some of the difficulties."[15]

In view of the hesitancy of the government, the proposal was modified and a request made for support for an initial period of five years only with no commitment beyond that time. The government was asked to give $5000 to renovate Queen's Hall, a university building that had fallen into disuse, and an additional $1000 toward the furnishings. On 30 May 1932, support was given to the extent of making the building available, with the understanding that training in public health nursing and hospital management would be carried on.[16] The Rockefeller Foundation gave an appropriation of $85,000 for the five-year period. The statute establishing the School was enacted by the Senate of the university on 10 June 1933, and the first classes were enrolled in the fall of that year.

As one would anticipate, financial difficulties beset the new School. However, income from students' fees, together with the support of the university and the Rockefeller Foundation, made possible the continuation and expansion of the programme.* Encouragement was given by the Rockefeller Foundation when the president referred to the progress made by the School: "In the early thirties aid was given to the School of Nursing of the University of Toronto, to establish a basic professional programme in the preparation of students for community nursing service. Kathleen Russell's leadership, scholarly ability and insight into the community's nursing needs have produced an outstanding research programme, and Toronto is one of the peaks of nursing training in the world."[17]

When the work of the School expanded well beyond the capacity of the old building at 7 Queen's Park, the foundation appropriated $300,000 toward the cost of a new building, bringing the total foundation support to $661,000. In the thirty-year period ending in 1953, the Foundation supported the development of nursing education in 48 schools in 28 countries. The University of Toronto was the only Canadian university to receive this support.

In addition to supporting the School, the foundation contributed to the development of public health training facilities for medical and nursing students. In 1939 the foundation gave a grant of $20,000 to the School of Hygiene which was matched by the Ontario government. This made possible the development of a suburban health department as a university teaching field. The School of Nursing was invited to name a senior nurse to be jointly appointed to the School and the health department. The association of the School of Nursing with this development enriched its field-work facilities, and contributed to the maintenance of a close relationship with the School of Hygiene and with a health department that was able to establish a high quality of service and to contribute to the School's teaching and research programme.

THE FACULTY OF THE SCHOOL

In the initial period following the establishment of the Department of Public Health Nursing, Kathleen Russell was fortunate in

* The interest and assistance of the President of the University, Dr. H. J. Cody, and the Director of the School of Hygiene, Dr. J. G. Fitzgerald, and a number of colleagues in the School of Hygiene and the Faculty of Medicine contributed to the success achieved during this critical period.

securing as her assistant a colleague with whom she had been associated in the Toronto Department of Public Health. Florence Emory
had just completed special preparation for public health nursing at
Simmons College, Boston, when in 1925 she accepted the position
of associate director, a position she held for over thirty years.

With the founding of the School in 1933, a challenge that faced
the director and her associate was the recruitment of staff qualified
to introduce innovations in nursing education, and to teach basic students and graduates of the diploma schools. Among the criteria
established for faculty positions were: the capacity for independent
and creative thought and critical analysis, a broad concept of nursing, a university degree representing sound, general education in the
humanities, and preparation for teaching.[18] As nurses with these
qualifications were difficult to find, fellowships were secured to assist
those selected to undertake additional study and to broaden their
understanding of nursing through travel and observation in other
countries. Fellowships were also sought for nursing service personnel who were associated with the School in the development of the
clinical resources for teaching.

A strong group of nursing educators was recruited. These women
recognized the need for reform in nursing education and were willing
to cast their lot with the School despite its tenuous financial position.
Their faith proved to be well-founded. Many had challenging lifetime careers in nursing education with the satisfaction that comes to
those who engage in the "imaginative consideration of learning."[19]
In addition to their contribution to the School, these staff members
served as officers in the professional associations and as board members of various community health agencies. Through this work they
increased their opportunities to interpret their educational philosophy and the goals they held for nursing to colleagues in the health
professions, and to gain the support of these colleagues and of interested citizens.

1933: THE FIRST BASIC COURSE

The primary purpose of the School when it was established in 1933
was to undertake a special study of the education and training of the
public health nurse.[20] It was inevitable that this should lead to an
examination of the general training for nursing. A thirty-nine month

basic course was developed in which content in the health and curative aspects of nursing was related so that the graduates would qualify for employment in any field of practice. Content in the biological and social sciences was provided by appropriate university departments. The faculty of the School were responsible for the classroom and clinical teaching of nursing; experiences were arranged in co-operation with the Toronto General Hospital and other selected hospitals and health agencies.

The unique characteristic of the School was its independence from the hospital. No other Canadian school of nursing had financial freedom and control over the students during periods of clinical experience and practice. Nursing education and nursing service were for the first time established as two interrelated but distinct entities, each administered independently of the other.

The hospitals co-operated with the School and contributed to the education of the students by permitting the faculty to select experiences for the students and to teach them in the clinical setting. During these clinical experiences the students accepted responsibility for the nursing care of the patients and for carrying out the policies of the particular hospital. The faculty of the School remained with the students, guiding their learning experiences and helping them to relate theory to practice. The Toronto General Hospital gave generous assistance and support to the programme. Indeed, so close a relationship developed that at one time consideration was given to the possibility of merging the two schools.

RESIDENCE LIFE: A RICH EDUCATIONAL EXPERIENCE

It was traditional at this time for student nurses to live in residence and the university followed this pattern. In keeping with this tradition, the director and faculty shared residence life with the students. This was a rich educational experience, as Kathleen Russell believed that young women could not be adequately prepared for such a personal type of service as nursing if they lived dully and unimaginatively.[21]

An atmosphere of mutual respect and concern for others permeated the residence. Despite budgetary restrictions, meals were attractive and service was generous. After-dinner coffee was served in a large living room with a fire-place in which a bright fire burned on winter evenings. This social hour provided the opportunity for stimulating conversation and the exchange of ideas. The students, many of whom came from distant lands, met the director, faculty, and guests of the School in an informal setting. Among the visitors were scholars and eminent persons representative of many fields including music, theology, and science as well as the professions. Holidays and other special occasions were marked by suitable festivities. No trouble was spared to transform the old rooms at 7 Queen's Park and to enlarge the dining area so that the students and their guests could enjoy the hospitality of the School. The need for recreation and between-meal snacks was met by a small basement room, affectionately known as the "bassinette," which was furnished as a student lounge.

A committee of faculty and students met at regular intervals to consider regulations and other matters that affected residence life. Kathleen Russell met the needs of the students with insight, generosity, and a sense of humour. When she was awakened late one night by a student coming in a basement window she apologized to the student for her having been obliged to enter by the window rather than the front door. The student was assured that in future, regardless of the hour, she should ring the door-bell. Later, when Miss Russell herself was locked out, she discovered that the bell did not arouse the sleepers within. A new bell was installed to ensure that anyone ringing at night would be heard.

As these were "depression" years, it was difficult to secure funds for the residence. Kathleen Russell often drew upon her personal resources so that residence life could be shared by as many as possible and hospitality could be extended to the students' guests. She furnished and maintained an apartment in a building nearby to provide additional accommodation. This apartment became home for many students from distant countries. Residence life was a rare and meaningful experience long remembered by these students.

THE APPEAL FOR STANDARDS

During the period in which the School was developing the diploma course, other universities in Canada and the United States were introducing degree programmes. These programmes had many of the undesirable features of the four-year diploma course discontinued at Toronto in 1933. Kathleen Russell believed the first objective of a university school of nursing should be to gain control over the conditions of clinical teaching and practice in the hospitals. Until this control was secured, she thought it would be impossible to meet the standards of the university. "If the degree is of uncertain value (she wrote) will it be worth our while *just at present*, to sacrifice anything of more certain value for it? Is it wise at the present time to ignore the degree, temporarily at least, and to concentrate upon the desired content and method of our nursing courses?"[22]

To encourage women with a broad liberal education to enter nursing, a special arrangement of the diploma course was provided for graduates of the Faculty of Arts. The academic background of these students made possible a strengthening of the nursing content, together with a reduction in the length of the course. The students who completed this arrangement had a strong academic and professional education on which to base nursing practice and later postgraduate work.[23]

THE CONTRIBUTION OF THE SCHOOL TO DIPLOMA EDUCATION

In addition to these courses the School made an extensive contribution to diploma education. An opportunity was provided for students enrolled in the Toronto schools to attend a series of lectures in public health nursing during the period in which they were assigned to community health agencies. In order to help the students to apply this experience the hospitals were encouraged to add to their staffs an instructor qualified in public health nursing.

A wide variety of refresher courses was offered to assist graduate nurses to add to their knowledge in specialized areas. The certificate courses were expanded to include clinical supervision, teaching, and administration of hospital and public health nursing service. Special programmes were arranged for individual students interested in more advanced work.

During this period many nurses from distant lands came to study at the School. Between 1917 and 1951, the Rockefeller Foundation awarded 476 fellowships to nurses, of which 197 were sent to Toronto, the largest number to attend any one university school of nursing. Other international and national agencies also sponsored students for study abroad. As a result, the School's influence was extended to over sixty countries in all regions of the world. Initially the majority of these students came from Europe. As the various countries expanded their health services, and sponsoring agencies became interested in contributing to these developments, students came from other regions including Oceania, North, South, and Central America, the West Indies, Asia, and Africa. Special programmes were arranged for some, and others completed one of the degree or certificate courses. These fellowship students were carefully selected for their ability and potential, and many have exerted leadership in the development of nursing and health services in their homelands.

1942: THE FIRST DEGREE COURSE

With experience gained in the diploma course, the faculty turned to the development of a degree course in nursing. The distinctive feature of this course was the integration of the general education subjects with the more specialized professional subject matter. A curriculum was planned in which content in the humanities and sciences was related to nursing in each year of the course. A careful selection from general education resulted in a balance in the humanities and the social and biological sciences, with a sequence of subjects in the three areas. Content in general education was related to nursing with the objective of adding to and enriching the learning in each area. The faculty of the School accepted responsibility for teaching nursing in the classroom and the clinical fields. The health and social implications of nursing were considered as essential in the preparation of the practitioner as was the care and rehabilitation of the sick. Throughout the course, consideration was given to the prevention of illness and the promotion of health, and experiences were arranged in a number of community health and social agencies in addition to those arranged in the general and specialized hospitals.

Excerpts from the writings of Kathleen Russell and her colleague, Jean Wilson, illustrate the philosophy held by the faculty:

The intention is to prepare professional women who, through studies of the humanities and sciences, will grow in understanding and wisdom;

with this education in the realm of human values, they may approach with safety the work that is awaiting them. ... Obviously, this preparation will include a sound scientific basis. We wish to combine the technical with the general subjects throughout the whole University course, believing that the richer results will be obtained by this method.[24]

The student is in the ward to acquire the art of nursing ... the student will learn that nursing is good only when it is good for the patient and when it gives service as broad in scope as the patient needs ... [the] instructor will make sure that her student has an ever-increasing appreciation of the patient; and that she grows daily in the sympathy for, and sensitiveness to, his needs that mark the fine flowering of the art of nursing.[25]

... as a learner [the student] passes from the classroom to the patient's bedside in the ward, from hospital ward to a practice field in some community health service, thence back to the classroom or seminar table, or library, and so on in unbroken progress through all the closely-knit study and practice from which she derives excellence in the art of nursing ... the important feature of this concept is the mobility of both student and instructor.[26]

... this instructor will use every opportunity that her clinical teaching offers to illustrate and illuminate the academic studies of her pupils: humanistic and social studies can be vitalized through this contact with patients. At the same time, patient care itself can be enriched by the greater insight afforded by these same studies.[27]

Initially the degree course was offered only to basic students. Graduates of the diploma schools were encouraged to enrol in the Faculty of Arts and to add to their programme of studies the nursing content of one of the certificate courses. Following three academic years they could qualify for the BA degree and a certificate in a nursing specialty. This arrangement was unsatisfactory as some of the "deepest values" of a full university education in nursing could not be achieved in this "disconnected type of preparation."[28]

Although this difficulty could not be overcome, a post-basic degree course was developed in 1952. This course provided an opportunity for study in the humanities, social sciences, and nursing. In 1965 the curriculum was revised so that more of the values of the basic course could be offered to diploma-school graduates. An integrated course was planned with content in the humanities and social

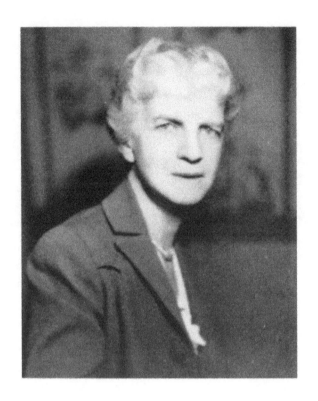

Edith Kathleen Russell, founder of the
University of Toronto School of Nursing

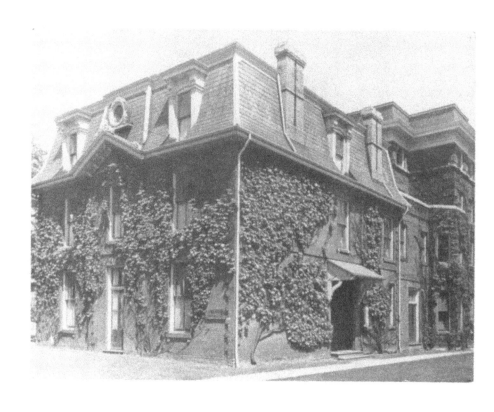

The old School of Nursing, 7 Queen's Park, occupied from 1933 to 1952

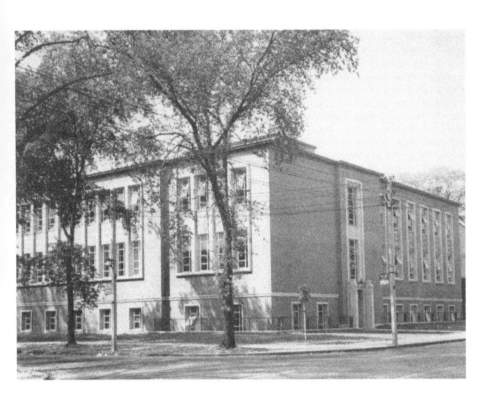

The present School of Nursing, built in 1952

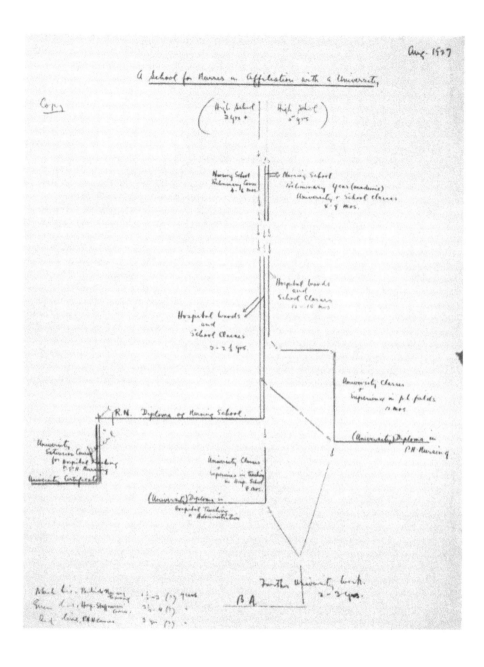

Chart illustrating Miss Russell's first plan for a new approach to nursing education. From a drawing by Miss Russell.

and biological sciences related to nursing in each year. The nursing subjects provided an opportunity for the students to broaden and increase their understanding of the preventive and curative aspects of nursing, and to focus on the individual needs of patients and their families. Study in the two functional areas, teaching and administration, was also included. Provision was made for the students to complete the subjects of the first and second years on a part-time basis in the Division of Extension as an alternative to three academic years of full-time study.

During the twenty-five years since the first baccalaureate degree course was introduced, the demand for this type of preparation has increased. At present the demand is so great that less than 50 per cent of the qualified applicants to the basic course can be accepted. Students with a strong motivation toward nursing and high academic standing seek admission. In the 1968–69 session, seventy-seven students were enrolled in the basic course, of whom 42 per cent had class I standing in Grade 13 and 51 per cent, class II standing.

Accompanying the increase in the degree courses has been an annual decrease in enrolment in the certificate courses from nearly 200 between 1945 and 1955 to approximately 100 ten years later, when the decision was made to phase out this work. Three of the four certificate courses that were offered in 1965 have now been discontinued. The public health nursing course will be continued for an interim period pending a decision concerning the need for the course and the most suitable location for the preparation of diploma graduates for this work.

THE YEARS AHEAD

The approach of a fiftieth anniversary is an occasion to evaluate the present as well as to reflect on the past. Critical analysis is an essential aspect of planning. An examination of current trends and developments is an aid to the formulation of guidelines for the future.

Advances in the medical sciences and the expansion of the health services have led to fundamental changes in health care. New patterns for the delivery of the health services have an impact on nursing. The baccalaurate courses must be kept under constant review to ensure that content and method of teaching remain relevant in the light of these advances.

A revision of the basic course was introduced in 1968. The major change was in the teaching of nursing which is being presented in each of the four years as a core subject consisting of the knowledge, skills, and attitudes applicable to the practice of nursing in any situation. Minor modifications were made in the humanities and sciences. These are arranged in the first, second, and third years, with a sequence provided in each area.

In the first year the focus in nursing is on normal growth and development. Students learn to assess patient needs as the first step in the nursing process, and to gain an understanding of the health services and personnel who contribute to these services, with particular attention to the role of the nurse. In the second and third years the study of the nursing process is continued with application to maternal-infant, medical-surgical (child and adult), and psychiatric nursing. Students have the opportunity for experience in caring for a variety of patients and families at different points on the health-illness continuum. A comprehensive nursing experience is planned in which the student can follow a family through all stages of an illness whether the care be provided by a hospital or by some other community health service. The whole of the fourth year is devoted to nursing to permit the students to concentrate on their major subject and to gain experience in the application of their knowledge in a variety of settings. An opportunity is provided in this year for independent study and individually planned experiences.

The over-all objectives of the basic and post-basic courses are the same. These courses provide the educational base for leadership in the provision of nursing care in hospitals and other health agencies, for administration of nursing service, and for teaching in schools of nursing. The content and general approach are similar although not identical.

The students who enrol in the post-basic course are a heterogeneous group, representative of a number of schools, a broad range of experience, and different levels of maturity. In the general education subjects common to both courses, the basic and post-basic students are in the same classes, and, where appropriate, grouped with students in other courses in the university. The nursing subjects, with one exception, are planned and arranged separately. This policy may be modified when the basic course curriculum revision is more fully implemented, and the faculty have additional experience in teaching nursing to the two groups of students. It would be helpful if an examination could be given to the graduate nursing students on admission to the university to test their knowledge and skills. If an accurate assessment could be made, electives might be offered to meet the students' needs. Alternatively, the post-basic students might be placed in selected nursing subjects with the basic students.

Diploma-school graduates with interest in and ability for university work should be encouraged to enrol in a university nursing course, as nurses with this preparation are needed for positions in service and education. When the basic baccalaureate courses have expanded to the point at which the universities can admit all the qualified applicants, the demand for the degree course for graduates of diploma schools of nursing should decrease. The students who have qualification for university education should take their initial preparation for nursing in the basic course. This would assure a sounder preparation, more efficient use of the university's resources, and a more economical use of the student's time. The needs of the diploma-school graduates who later become interested in a university education for nursing could probably be met within the basic course.

In order for the undergraduate courses to thrive and for the School to continue to give leadership in nursing, graduate education should be developed. Nursing has become broader in scope and nurses have begun to assume responsibilities of greater complexity. There is a need for nurses with a depth of knowledge beyond that attainable in a baccalaureate course. These nurses will participate in patient care in specialized clinical areas and contribute to the advancement of nursing knowledge and skills through analytical study and investigation. They will also fill senior positions in administration, consultation, and teaching. The development of graduate education should have high priority as "It is in graduate studies that the complementary aspects of teaching and research are most pronounced ... [Graduate studies] offer the surest guarantee of transmitting into undergraduate teaching, the excitement and discovery characterizing the progress of knowledge in whatever branch it may be. ... Graduate studies, in truth, underpin undergraduate instruction just as they overarch it."[29]

The School should accept responsibility for the development of a continuing education programme to meet the needs of university nursing graduates. These nurses must be kept informed of innovations and abreast of advances in nursing. They need the opportunity to up-date their knowledge and skills in hospital and community nursing practice, teaching, and administration. Evaluation and research are important aspects of continuing education to which the school should make a contribution.

A trend can be discerned with regard to the organization of health sciences faculties and schools to facilitate the sharing of certain resources, the interchange of ideas, and the development of new educational opportunities for the students. Technological advances have an impact on administration and education and new and expensive equipment should be shared by units that have common interest and needs.

Students have become interested in participating in policy-making bodies that affect their education and welfare. This is a relatively new development, which is worthy of study. Experience to date indicates that nursing students can make a valuable contribution to certain committees such as those concerned with the library, the curricula, and financial aid. An extension of student participation to other areas may be desirable. The time students can give is limited because of the pressures of a professional education in which there is clinical experience as well as course work. The interest of students in university affairs should be fostered and students encouraged to continue to take an active interest in their Alma Mater through membership in the Alumni Association following graduation.

THE SCHOOL: AN AGENT OF CHANGE

Throughout the years, the University of Toronto School of Nursing has been looked upon as a laboratory for the study of educational problems in nursing. From the outset an interest has been taken in the diploma schools, as well as in university nursing education. Kathleen Russell made a significant contribution to the study of nursing education at the diploma level through her participation in the Joint Committee responsible for the *Survey of Nursing Education in Canada*.[30] Nettie Fidler, the second director, conducted the demonstration of diploma education at the Metropolitan School of Nursing in Windsor. The findings of this study were widely discussed and influenced the pattern of diploma education in North America.[31]

Through experience in teaching public health nursing, the faculty became interested in enriching the content of the diploma programmes. As early as 1945, Kathleen Russell envisaged the diploma schools as being able to prepare a nurse who could be "accepted officially as an assistant to the public health nurse."[32] Now the School is urging an examination and evaluation of the curricula in these schools to ascertain the extent to which the health and preventive aspects of nursing can be included in these programmes. The time may have come to implement the recommendations made in 1945. Diploma schools may be able to prepare nurses to serve as members of the nursing team in hospitals and other community health agencies with graduates of the degrees courses serving as team leaders. If this should prove to be a feasible and economical approach in the delivery of public health nursing service, the certificate course in public health nursing would no longer be needed.

The School has also influenced the development of university nursing education in Canada and abroad. Programmes developed along the lines of those at Toronto have been established in nineteen universities in Canada.

Contributions have been made by the faculty through research and writing. Briefs have been submitted to the Royal Commission on Health Services and the Committee on the Healing Arts in Ontario. In the brief to the Royal Commission the faculty recommended that diploma programmes be developed within the framework of education, the exact place within the educational system to be established by research. As a result of this recommendation, the Registered Nurses' Association of Ontario sponsored a demonstration programme at the Ryerson Institute of Technology in Toronto.

Through its graduates, the School has extended its influence in nursing across Canada and throughout the world. The Alumni Association, now numbering nearly 5000, has given strong support to the School. The bursary programme developed by the alumni has contributed to the recruitment and financial support of able students. Fund-raising activities made possible the inclusion of Cody Hall* in the School, a large auditorium widely used by professional and educational bodies within the university and the community.

A survey has been made of the contribution of the graduates of

---

* This auditorium was named in honour of Dr. H. J. Cody, president and Chancellor of the University of Toronto, 1932–47. Mrs. Cody, a graduate of the class of 1921, was the first president of the Alumnae Association.

the basic course in the twenty-year period from 1946 to 1966. Of the 446 graduates, 294 replied to mailed questionnaires. Forty-five per cent of the respondents were active in nursing at the time the questionnaire was completed. Seventy-three per cent of those who graduated between 1962 and 1966 were employed in nursing. Fifty-six per cent had at some time held positions in education, administration, or research. Approximately one-half belonged to their professional organization, and over one-half were active in community affairs; nearly three-quarters of those not actively engaged in nursing were associated with some form of community service. Frustrations in the work situation most frequently reported were due to factors preventing good nursing care. In many cases the graduates felt unable to influence nursing care in such a way as to put into practice the values and ideals they had learned.[33]

In an address to the Alumni Association shortly after it was organized, Kathleen Russell said "... for it is to you members of the Alumnae Association that we look for leadership of the future. The only unforgiveable sin consists of inaction, unwillingness to do anything at all. The greatest teacher and philosopher of all time left us this lesson in the parable of the talents. The man who was utterly condemned was the careful, fearful one who hid his talent away and did nothing."[34]

Kathleen Russell was in truth a dynamic realist. Her imaginative insight largely determined the goals of the School, yet their achievement was shared by many: a challenging student body, a vital Alumni Association, understanding colleagues from a variety of disciplines, and a strong and able staff. Kathleen Russell guided and motivated students and faculty through her keen intellect, her commitment to nursing, and her dedication to the goals of the School. In turn she sought support and counsel from those around her. She encouraged the faculty in their teaching and gave great freedom to them to contribute to the community and the organized profession. Already the expanding School enjoys a wide sphere of influence, but for assessment, the full impact of its work awaits the unfolding years.

In a tribute paid to Miss Russell at the time of her death, Florence Emory, her close associate for nearly thirty years, wrote "It has been said that greatness is attained through changing the course of events and changing them for always. If this be true, then in retrospect there can be detected in Edith Kathleen Russell's professional life and work an element of true greatness."[35]

NOTES

1 The Canadian Red Cross Society, "The Role of One Voluntary Organization in Canada's Health Services," A Brief Presented to the Royal
Commission on Health Services, 1962, p. 14.
2 University of Toronto, *School of Nursing Calendar, 1933–34*, p. 7.
3 E. Kathleen Russell, "The Teaching of Public Health Nursing in the
University of Toronto," reprinted from *Methods and Problems of Medical
Education*, twenty-first series (New York, 1932), p. 2.
4 E. MacPherson Dickson, "Report of the Inspector of Training Schools
in the Province of Ontario," 1923, p. 1.
5 *Ibid.*, p. 3.
6 Report of the Committee, *Nursing and Nursing Education in the United
States* (New York, 1923).
7 E. Kathleen Russell, "The Relation of Nurse Education to the University
of Toronto," Typewritten memorandum, 15 August 1927, p. 2.
8 *Ibid.*, p. 3.
9 Mary Beard, *The Nurse in Public Health* (New York, 1929), p. 210.
10 E. Kathleen Russell, "Concerning the Training of a Public Health Nurse,"
memorandum attached to a letter addressed to Dr. J. G. Fitzgerald,
Director, School of Hygiene, 16 May 1932.
11 E. Kathleen Russell, "University of Toronto School of Nursing, Progress
Report," 31 December 1934, p. 4.
12 Letter to Mary Beard, 29 November 1929.
13 E. Kathleen Russell, "The Teaching of Public Health Nursing in the
University of Toronto," p. 6.
14 Letter to Dr. A. Primrose, Dean of the Faculty of Medicine, 15 November
1930.
15 Letter to the Honourable George S. Henry, Prime Minister of Ontario,
9 September 1931.
16 Letter to Kathleen Russell from the Honourable George S. Henry, 30
May 1932.
17 Raymond B. Fosdick, *The Rockefeller Foundation Annual Report, 1947*,
p. 30.
18 E. Kathleen Russell, "Regarding Staff (or Faculty Members) of a University School of Nursing," June 1948, p. 1.
19 Alfred North Whitehead, *The Aims of Education* (New York, 1949),
p. 97.
20 University of Toronto, *School of Nursing Calendar, 1933–34*, p. 7.
21 "University of Toronto School of Nursing, Progress Report," p. 1.
22 E. Kathleen Russell, "Canadian Universities and Canadian Schools of
Nursing," *Canadian Nurse* XXIV (December 1928): 630.
23 University of Toronto, *School of Nursing Calendar, 1940–41*, p. 8.
24 E. Kathleen Russell, "Fifty Years of Medical Progress, Medicine as a
Social Instrument: Nursing," *New England Journal of Medicine* CCXLIV
(22 March 1951): 444.
25 E. Kathleen Russell and M. Jean Wilson, "Nursing Education – Methods
of Clinical Instruction," *Canadian Nurse* XLV (November 1949): 823–4.
26 *Ibid.*, p. 821.
27 *Ibid.*, p. 825.
28 *Ibid.*, p. 822.
29 Report of the President's Committee on the School of Graduate Studies,

Graduate Studies in The University of Toronto (Toronto, 1965), pp. 16–17.

30 George W. Weir, *Survey of Nursing Education in Canada* (Toronto, 1932), p. 581.

31 A. R. Lord, *Report of the Evaluation of the Metropolitan School of Nursing* (Windsor, Ont., 1952), p. 54.

32 E. Kathleen Russell, "Request for Financial Aid toward a New Building," Report Prepared for the International Health Division, Rockefeller Foundation, 7 March 1945, p. 4.

33 Nora I. Parker, *Survey of Graduates of the University of Toronto Baccalaureate Course in Nursing* (School of Nursing, University of Toronto, 1968), p. 44.

34 Bulletin from the Alumnae Association of the Department of Public Health Nursing, University of Toronto, 1931 and 1932, p. 3.

35 Florence H. M. Emory, *Edith Kathleen Russell, An Appreciation of Her Professional Life and Work* (School of Nursing, University of Toronto, 6 March 1964), p. 4.

6
The development of nursing education at the diploma level

BLANCHE DUNCANSON

Nursing lore is as old as mankind and with few exceptions has been associated with the traditional nurturing role performed by the female as she cared for members of her family. Those who developed special skills in the areas of childbirth and care of the sick, injured, or dying were designated by their families and neighbours to either perform these skills as the need arose or transfer their knowledge to other members of the family to provide for its dissemination to succeeding generations.

The development of the Christian church in western civilization, with its attendant organizations and institutions, provided a vehicle whereby females could be of service to their fellow men in pursuit of their religious vocation. The Christian traditions of charity, devotion, dedication, respect, and love for one's fellow man found a ready application in the service of the sick and poor, the abandoned, the persecuted, and the disadvantaged.

These traditions reached the shores of Canada through the influence of the Jesuits. Wealthy and powerful in their own right, the Jesuits tried to rouse the court of France to a sense of religious and political obligations in Quebec, and to awaken the nobility and rich bourgeoisie to a realization of the opportunities for pious benefactions and self-sacrifice in the new world. The schools and hospitals at Quebec and Montreal, the Indian villages at Sillery and Three Rivers and all the chief foundations of the period can be traced directly or indirectly to the work of the Jesuits.[1]

The Hotel Dieu of Quebec owes its inception to the interest created in France by the published *Relations* (reports) made by the first Jesuit missionaries to New France.[2] One who was moved to action was the Duchess d'Aiguillon, a niece of Cardinal Richelieu. Inspired by the Gospel of Charity, she founded the Hotel Dieu at Quebec in 1639 with the assistance of the Augustinian Hospitallers of Dieppe. These sisters were bound by vow to the cloister, celibacy, poverty, obedience, and care of the sick. A similar background prevailed for the Hospitallers of St. Joseph of La Flèche who took over Jeanne Mance's Hotel Dieu at Montreal. Gradually the French-born sisters were outnumbered and were eventually replaced by the Canadian-born nurses.

The sisters' courage, serenity, and devotion never wavered under the most adverse circumstances – lack of supplies, pestilence, rigours of weather, epidemics of typhus, influenza, smallpox, and scurvy, and danger from the Iroquois. Their true temper was tested by the British attack on New France and the ultimate capitulation of Quebec in 1759. "These Sisters provided a liaison between French and English which made it easier to lay the foundations for a United Canada."[8]

From the influence of the early sisters have developed some of the most charitable concepts found in the care and cure of the ill and in the very important field of prevention and health teaching. The expansion of religious hospitals and the development of lay hospitals in the nineteenth century were the result of society's concern and efforts to cope with the ravages of illness due to epidemics, the high incidence of injuries, and wounds resulting from military exploits or the vicissitudes of life in a virgin country which appeared inimical to human habitation.

Any reference to lay nurses between 1750 and 1800 is sporadic and it can be assumed that their services were voluntary and that their preparation for the service was a compound of intuitive sensitivity about and devotion to the needs of others, knowledge acquired through practice and the use of skills and remedies that had been found effective by themselves or other nurses, with whom they might have served as apprentices.

As the practice of medicine emerged as a skilful professional service, physicians added to the nurses' ability by individual or group instruction. In the early nineteenth century, benevolent societies and volunteer nurses complemented the sisterhoods' activities in attempting to deal with the problems of destitute families affected by war and of destitute immigrants plagued with disease and debilitation from the long sea voyage almost totally devoid of sanitary precautions. Their efforts accompanied the colonists as they pushed west from Montreal and Quebec to Upper Canada and to the prairie regions.

Under the British North America Act, among the powers assigned to the provinces were education, health, and welfare. The provinces did not immediately exercise their rights in health matters, since the development of hospitals had followed a pattern of "voluntarism" in control and financing. This meant that the development of hospitals was subject to the philanthropic and humanitarian characteristics of individuals in society and reflected the needs of society as society perceived them. With the advances in medical science and the improvements in medical education, the place of the hospital in advancing health care was recognized by the medical profession and by society at large. The desire of all classes of society for active treatment necessitated revision in the hospitals' policies in respect to accessibility to both the indigent patient and the patient able to defray in part or *in toto* the cost of hospitalization. The best care possible consistent with a cost that did not exploit illness became a guiding principle in hospital operations.

Society believed that a large proportion of care should be provided by the newly emerging trained nurse. It had been demonstrated by Florence Nightingale that nurses who were trained in the skills of observing, recording, and reporting of data pertinent to a patient's condition, in providing comfort and therapeutic measures, and in the development of personal traits of devotion, dedication, and compassion improved the quality of care for hospital patients. It was natural that a country so young as Canada should look to the example afforded by this pioneer in nursing education for a solution to the increasing needs of physicians and patients for trained personnel to assist them.

The Nightingale School of Nursing associated with St. Thomas's Hospital, London, England, came into being in 1860 through the inspiration and guidance of Florence Nightingale. A fund established in her honour for her work in the Crimean War was used to defray the costs of establishing and operating this school. This money was entirely separate from and formed no part of the hospital's budget and, administered as it was by the Nightingale Fund Council, it did not come under the control of the voluntary board of the hospital. This gave the Council freedom of action, subject only to approval by Florence Nightingale, to establish the financial and training policies of the school. As this system was transferred to Canada and the United States, the concept of autonomy in the administration of financial and educational matters was lost. The schools of nursing became completely dependent on the financial stability of the hospital with which they were associated and their policies were formulated by a voluntary board appointed to administer the hospital. This pattern of organization and administration has led to innumerable problems in administering the educational preparation of nursing practitioners. Most importantly perhaps, the essential component of learning to provide nursing care, with accompanying practice, was subordinated to the service needs of the institution.

By 1900, twenty hospital training schools had been established in the major towns and cities of Canada. This number had increased to seventy by 1909.[4] Certain principles inherent in the first Nightingale School were inherent in these new schools. Women, as well prepared in nursing as the times allowed, were placed in charge of the schools. Courses were spread over a long period of time, two to three years. A modicum of incidental instruction was accompanied by extended periods of practice, but in an apprenticeship pattern that lacked the "master craftsman." One or two hours of lecture per week, given by a physician or the superintendent, was attended by those students who did not otherwise have responsibilities to care for patients in the clinical departments at the time. These students procured the information and transmitted it to their confrères who were unable to attend.

The recruitment of students into the early programmes did not present extreme difficulty. This was due in part to the quality of leaders who emerged and to the natural desire of young women to have a respectable career outside the home. Nursing's respectability was due to the efforts of the early leaders who moulded the "profession of nursing." The hospital's nursing care had to be made safe for both the patient and the student; patients with highly communicable disease – tuberculosis, in particular, were segregated from other patients. Obstructions, such as the distrust of the "nurses" who were without training and of some physicians who feared the nurses would take over medical duties, had to be overcome. A balance had to be found between the utilization of students over long hours in practical service to the hospital's patients and their required attendance in a programme of instruction. Hospital boards valued the students' services since they contributed to quality care at a surprisingly low cost – an important feature in the financial operation of voluntary public hospitals.

Little emphasis has been placed upon the efforts of the superintendents of nurses to upgrade the quality of the nurses' preparation, except in the annals of the professional organizations' records and reports. The superintendent has been cast in the role of an authoritarian figure, demanding deference and obedience while meting out stern discipline. With nursing's inherited traditions of military discipline and religious asceticism, with socety's attitude toward women in the Victorian era, and with the obstructions and doubts to be overcome, would it have been possible for the superintendent of nurses to develop a different role model? She had to face and solve problems without the aid of any precedent, colleague collaboration, or professional organization support.

Many of the working conditions for nurses when schools began to evolve were particularly unattractive and had a way of weaving themselves into school policies. Leaders had to concern themselves with reducing the students' workday (from 7:00 AM to 10:00 PM) to a twelve-hour period and then to a twelve-hour day with two hours off per day exclusive of time allowed for meals which were provided in a setting away from the ward. Regular class admissions were organized in lieu of admitting one student as another completed her programme. Formal instruction was organized with the aid of physicians but without the benefit of nurses who were qualified teachers. Teaching facilities were developed. Dormitories were converted to residences where a degree of privacy and recreation could be obtained, where social graces could be enhanced, and where students could be cared for in a manner consistent with parental and social expectations. All these tasks the leaders were required to accomplish in a society that did not uniformly educate its female members, or admit them to institutions of higher learning, or entitle them to exercise a franchise. At all times, the superintendent was required to be above reproach, as were her nurses. To depart from this state of grace was to commit an unpardonable social misdemeanour.

While great community pride reflected itself in its hospital and training school, it was the superintendent of nurses who identified the conflict in the priorities of each. The educational needs of the students were being subordinated to the nursing needs of the patients. With this dilemma she struggled in isolation, since she was held responsible both for the nursing service to the patients and for the education of the nursing students, and frequently for the administration of the hospital as well. In proportion to the superintendent's imbued conscientiousness, the conflict became more acute and ultimately the imperative demands of the suffering patient had to take precedence. Thus the nursing needs of the patient and the educational needs of the student were placed in continuing conflict.

Nurses, upon graduation, were free to seek their own employment with the result that the private practice of nursing emerged as the predominant employment category. A few remained to teach in the training school and some found employment in hospitals without training schools.

Although the quality of nursing services was held in high esteem, there was not a comparable economic value placed upon such services. Most of the costs of operating hospitals including training schools was borne by the private patient who paid fees for service. The same patient, in general, engaged the services of a graduate nurse in private duty. Since nursing's ethical standards did not encourage exploitation of the ill for personal gain, the nurses' economic position was in direct opposition to the social prestige accorded her. In the area of social prestige, too, a peculiar anomaly existed. Since the majority of private practice was carried out in the homes of the "private patients," the nurse was considered as a semi-employee and semi-servant yet expected to provide a twenty to twenty-four hour professional service to her patient.

The marked proliferation of nursing schools to meet the nursing needs of hospital patients in the first quarter of the twentieth century is readily understood. The alacrity with which students entered the smallest and the largest of these single-discipline schools is less well understood in the context of today's society. However, opportunities for women to be gainfully employed outside the home were few by comparison with the employment opportunities that exist today. Long periods of apprenticeship with rigorous discipline were not the exception nor were long hours of work with low pay. In industry, 75 to 84 hours of work per week were not exceptional. In a very young country, long hours of hard work were associated with potential success. In this same context, idealism and altruism were influential. Then, too, out of the crisis and chaos of the global conflict of 1914–18, the nurse emerged as a heroine – unflinching, fearless, and tireless in the face of danger, but gentle, sympathetic, charitable, and a source of strength to her fellow man. The superintendents of nursing had sought to improve the schools and direct the fledgling nursing vocation on its road to professional status. Once their schools were operational, they met together to share mutual concerns and goals and to plan means of achieving them. This proved to be the genesis of a national voluntary nurses' organization in which all trained nurses were eligible for membership. Shortly after its incorporation in the early 1900s, this organization, now known as the Canadian Nurses' Association, took the step of publishing and distributing to membership a nursing journal which dealt with professional and technical matters. Through the journal and through meeting together, the nurses recognized that unity was essential if they were to achieve the goal of obtaining legislative controls over minimum standards of education and practice. The effectiveness of their efforts in supporting demands for provincial registration acts, while unaccustomed to political activity, may be judged by the fact that such legislation was introduced and enacted before female suffrage was universally achieved.

After 1918, there was an increased demand for nursing services in military establishments, in the expanding public health programmes, in the provincial sanatoria, and in hospitals without schools. But there were fewer students entering nursing. Why was this happening? A series of surveys revealed the fact that there were increasing employment opportunities for women and that students were disenchanted with the conditions under which they were being trained. Canada, because of its proximity to the United States, was affected by the literature emanating from that country. One of the first reports, *Nursing and Nursing Education in the United States*,[5] had quite profound influence since it addressed its enquiry to the foregoing question and its findings, based on scientific methods, were presented in a factual manner. Goldmark, the author, questioning the validity of the humanity-first principle taking precedence over nursing education, stated:

A different solution [for nursing education] might be found, the sick might be cared for without sacrificing the very object for which the training school exists, the education of new generations of nurses. When in addition, it appears that the sacrifice of education is actively defeating the aims of the school – alienating instead of arousing the devotion of students contributing to the decreases in the number of applicants, turning out nurses of ill-balanced, widely diverse training, unfitted to meet modern needs – then the sacrifice of education wears a very different aspect.[6]

A Canadian survey under the direction of George M. Weir, and co-sponsored by the Canadian Nurses' Association and the Canadian Medical Association, had as its aim the possible improvement of nursing education in Canada.[7] From the accumulated evidence gained during the survey, Weir asserted that "The state can establish no logical justification for permitting the cost [of training student nurses] to be charged to the cost of illness."[8] Some of the factors in the future education of the nurse expected to become actualities in the ensuing ten years were: "Abandonment of apprenticeship standards ..., and the adoption of ones more characteristic of real education as found ... in the modern, normal school or university ... From a financial viewpoint, nursing education should be made an integral part of the provincial educational system."[9]

Following the Weir survey, the Canadian Nurses' Association assessed the steps it would have to take to fulfil the survey recommendations. Believing that the establishment of nursing education on an independent financial basis and on a fully recognized professional level could only come about gradually, the Canadian Nurses' Association turned its attention to the establishment of a curriculum guide for schools of nursing as an immediate objective.[10] This guide pointed the way for improving nursing education through upgrading the qualifications of students and teachers, and by developing an integrated curriculum within a school organized on a sound administrative basis, with control of educational policies and "command of sufficient financial resources to provide the necessary facilities."[11] The curriculum guide was predicated on the belief that "schools of nursing in Canada will probably continue to be conducted under the administration and control of hospitals."[12]

The foregoing activities, accompanied by a rigorous recruiting programme, the provision and requirement of additional preparation for teachers, improvements in the educational training programme, and a relaxation of unnecessarily restrictive supervisory and disciplinary measures by the schools, led to a stop-gap solution. This solution, although subject to review during the years of the depression and shored up during the extreme demands for nursing during the Second World War, left nursing education in an extremely vulnerable and chaotic position in the second half of the twentieth century. The situation was similar to the one that followed the First World War. The problems were intensified in proportion to the rapid expansion in the demands for nursing services, to the backlog from the depression period when numbers of recruits were restricted and preparation for leadership was economically impossible for all but a very few, and to other opportunities which offered more social and economic security to prospective recruits.

The underlying causative factor in the diminution of recruits was not removed, namely the conflict caused by the priority which the hospital gave to its patients' service needs at the expense of providing the student with a liberal educational programme which would equip her to meet society's expanding health needs. To this factor was added the cumulative effect of the economic depression on nursing as a profession. Ethical platitudes were no longer sufficient, if indeed they ever were, to provide for the personal satisfaction and fulfilment of an individual's social needs as a nurse and as a citizen.

Throughout the foregoing period, the nursing profession made repeated representations to the government requesting public financial support for the education of nurses to be placed in institutions whose primary function was education. In recognition of the fact that nursing education's dilemma was only one facet of the problem faced by post-war governments attempting to provide economic security, social welfare, health services, and educational opportunities for the citizens, the nursing profession undertook to demonstrate its convictions in a positive, concrete manner.

A resolution at the Canadian Nurses' Association meeting in 1946 gave approval "to a demonstration being undertaken to determine whether a professional nurse can be prepared adequately in less than three years."[13] The immediate objectives of the demonstration carried out between 1948–52 were: "(a) to establish nursing schools as educational institutions, separate entities in their own right, and (b) to demonstrate, if possible, that a skilled clinical nurse can be prepared in a period shorter than three years, once the school is given control of the use of the students' time."[14]

The *Report of the Evaluation of the Metropolitan School of Nursing* was the first study in nursing undertaken in Canada since the

Weir survey.[15] The following quotation by Lord attests the success of the demonstration: "The conclusion is inescapable. When the school has complete control of students, nurses can be trained at least as satisfactorily in two years as in three and under better conditions, but the training must be paid for in money instead of in services. Few students can afford substantial fees nor can the hospital pass on such additional costs to the 'paying patient.' Some new source of revenue is the only solution."[16]

The Metropolitan Demonstration School was a successful demonstration, but duplication of this effort based on the principle of financial and administrative autonomy was not immediately forthcoming. The reasons for this can be attributed to society's traditional satisfaction with the precedence of training programmes under the administrative and financial control of hospitals – a system which led to varying degrees of excellence in schools which were essentially private in character, single-discipline in nature, devoid of the liberalizing components of a general education, and subject only to the outside influence of the standards for approval contained in the registration acts.

Referring to the system of nursing education with its concomitant confusion in priority of goals exposed and criticized in the Goldmark Report and the Weir Survey, Kathleen Russell stated:

Instead of radical change which might have taken place in the 1920's, we have worried through thirty additional years of confused effort, dealing with the symptoms, rather than the disease itself. Certainly some improvement in detail has been effected but the fundamental condition has remained the same in that the hospital board of governors pays for the school and therefore, controls it while the student has retained the status of an employee and works her passage through the training course by servicing the hospital. When the hospital has taken its responsibility for the students seriously the school has been a very expensive asset, and fortunately, the wisest hospitals are beginning to question the whole procedure.[17]

One hospital that questioned the whole procedure, even before the completion of the Metropolitan Demonstration School project, was the Toronto Western Hospital. A pilot project was undertaken in 1950 for a five-year period. The objectives of this project were twofold: to increase the number of recruits for the nursing profession and to improve the quality of nursing education in a hospital-owned school of nursing.[18] Following the example of the Metropolitan Demonstration School, control of the student-nurses' time for learning experiences, both classroom and clinical, in the first two years was vested in the school. At the end of this time, the student was entitled to write the registration examinations but then was required to spend a third or internship year in the hospital's nursing service before she was eligible for registration.

The fulfilment of the objectives of the pilot project was tested by comparing the results of the students' performance with preceding groups of students, in the same school, who had followed the more traditional three-year programme. A unique opportunity was afforded in 1952 when the same registration examinations were written by two classes of students in the same school. One class had completed the traditional three-year programme, and the second class had completed two years of the new programme. Following a review of the results, Stewart stated, "The figures show that the revised two-year course had produced, from the academic point of view, results far superior to the old three-year course."[19] In the matter of recruitment during the project period, Stewart noted that, "the rate of enrolment of students in the school had increased by twenty-five percent."[20]

In concluding his report, which referred also to the cost of educating a nurse, Stewart asked, "Is there any valid reason why the education of nurses should not receive from public funds the same support as is given to the education of engineers, architects, teachers, druggists, dentists and ... librarians?"[21]

As valuable as the demonstration projects were, the fact remained that little, if any, major revision was taking place in the total field of nursing education along the lines recommended in the Weir survey some twenty-five years previously. The Canadian Nurses' Association remained very concerned about its responsibility in maintaining a high level of nursing service. The Association studied the merits of the accreditation process and, after much deliberation on behalf of its 55,000 members, decided to conduct a "Pilot Project for the Evaluation of Schools of Nursing."[22] Such a project was designed to study all aspects of the accreditation procedure. National accreditation was perceived as a voluntary process whereby schools would apply for accreditation and be examined by the Canadian Nurses' Association. This body would evaluate and approve nursing schools on the basis of criteria that would be applied nationally and that would be developed nationally by the nursing profession. Other purposes of the project were as follows:

To determine the bases on which schools of nursing in Canada can be accredited.
To explore procedures for carrying out an accreditation program.
To determine the personnel and resources needed to carry out a national program of accreditation.
To estimate the cost of a national program of accreditation.
To acquaint the Canadian people with the needs of nursing.[23]

In the project, data were collected from twenty-five of the one hundred and seventy-four diploma schools in Canada. Evaluation of these data by a board of review revealed that the schools were not ready for a programme of accreditation, since 84 per cent of the schools surveyed did not meet the over-all quality suggested by the criteria which were used.

The director of study, Dr. Helen Mussallem, in compiling the recommendations gave priority to the following, namely, "that a re-examination of the whole field of nursing education be undertaken."[24] Mussallem pointed out that such a study "would be a comprehensive undertaking which would give consideration to the total health needs of the country and services required to meet them. It should consider the place of nursing in helping to meet these needs and suggest means of recruiting and preparing the necessary personnel. Such suggestions should be projected far enough into the future to give positive direction to the course of nursing."[25] This recommendation was to await the investigations of the Royal Commission on Health Services to be brought to fruition.

The prepaid hospital insurance scheme on a private and voluntary basis, and later sponsored and administered by provincial governments, was a major development in the late fifties. While this relieved the patient of the economic burden of hospitalization costs, the concomitant expansion of knowledge in the health services field, and consequently of services, increased the need for prepared personnel. The nursing profession decried the inclusion of the costs of nursing education in a system of prepaid hospital insurance made possible through the passage of the Hospital Insurance and Diagnostic Services Act. While it did not oppose the concept of prepaid hospital services insurance, the profession was opposed to the inclusion of the costs of operating a school of nursing in a service insurance programme. While the profession recognized it was "public support" for nursing education, the fundamental conflict, i.e., control of education by a service-oriented organization, was not being resolved. Katherine MacLaggan, the Chairman of the Committee on Nursing Education of the Canadian Nurses' Association, pinpointed the problem when she avowed:

The problem is not alone a financial one ... but [the] philosophy of nursing education is ... the important question. Some day, the people of this country must accept as a principle, open and public financial support of nursing education, in the same way that other forms of professional education are openly and publicly supported. ... The nursing profession needs the support of an informed public, in order to attach the student of nursing to a more suitable cost than the per diem rate for hospital service.[26]

The Royal Commission on Health Services in Canada was set up in 1961 by the Canadian government "to inquire into and report upon the existing facilities and the future need for health services for the people of Canada, the resources required to provide such services, and to recommend such measures, consistent with the constitutional division of legislative powers in Canada, as the Commissioners believe will ensure that the best possible health care is available to all Canadians."[27] A study of nursing education in Canada was requested by the Commission and was undertaken by Dr. Mussallem. The purpose of this study was to examine, describe, and analyse formal educational programmes for nurses and to make proposals for needed change.[28]

Among the significant recommendations emanating from this study are the following:

It was recommended that immediate plans should be directed towards introducing diploma schools of nursing into the post-high school system of the country. Until such time as an appropriate post-high school educational system evolved in Canada, e.g. Junior Community Colleges, it was suggested that the diploma schools be administratively under the aegis of a university. Then, to provide potential candidates for leadership positions sufficient recruits should be channelled into University Schools of Nursing. To provide candidates for leadership, at least twenty-five per cent of the candidates would need to be prepared in the University stream.[29]

Submissions from the provincial nurses' associations to the commission expressed convictions similar to those contained in the recommendations made by Mussallem. The belief was expressed that improvement in the quality, particularly the liberality of nursing education, was a necessary antecedent to upgrading the nature of nursing service. While the commissioners believed that placing nursing education under the control of educational authorities might be feasible, they were equally aware that the thirty years since the Weir survey "had tended to strengthen the hospital's financial and administrative control over nursing education."[30] The attendant weaknesses in this arrangement have been the emphasis on service which the student provides, the precedence which services take over the integration of classroom and clinical teaching, the low proportion of liberal education components, and the unnecessarily repetitive tasks that contribute little to learning but extend the length of time for the programme. Contributing to the weaknesses was a further complicating factor – an insufficient number of qualified teachers to provide the necessary instruction and supervision.

In view of the felt urgency to increase the number of nurses, the commission's recommendations dealt with the immediacy of the problems and suggested the following measures to immediately improve the quality of diploma education in the hospital schools:

1 That the budgets of the Schools of Nursing operated by hospitals be separated from that of the Nursing Service of the hospital to the end that the Schools of Nursing become wholly educational in their function.

2 That hospitals make their educational facilities available for the instruction and clinical experience of students, without claim on the student for service.

3 That the Schools of Nursing re-organize their curricula to provide for graduation, with a diploma in two years.[31]

However, in looking to the future supply of nurses, the commission emphasized "that a major effort must be made by governments, hospitals, the health professions, and the public if the education of nurses was to be integrated with higher education in general and if the quality of their education was to be improved."[32]

The commission predicted that between 1961 and 1971 "the supply of qualified nurses [in Canada] must increase by over 20,000 if present standards are maintained and could amount to nearly

42,000 if improved standards of patient care are provided" and that the annual output of university nursing graduates must increase several times to approach in 1971 the desired ratio of one university nurse to each three diploma nurses.[33]

During the hearings of the Royal Commission on Health Services, submissions made by the Canadian Nurses' Association, the Registered Nurses' Association of Ontario, and the School of Nursing, University of Toronto, contained the genesis of the concept which lead to the establishment of a nursing programme in the Ryerson Institute of Technology in Toronto.

In the brief submitted by the Canadian Nurses' Association, a new type of school was visualized. Such a school was to be "at the post-high school level, under the jurisdiction of institutions whose primary function is education."[34] Among the recommendations contained in the brief from the School of Nursing, University of Toronto, the opinion was expressed that nursing schools should be "established within the educational system of the province,"[35] that the exact place should be established by research, and that one type which might be investigated was a technological college.[36] In its submission, the Registered Nurses' Association of Ontario recommended "that the preparation of the nurse in a diploma programme be conducted within a general system of education"[37] and "that study be undertaken to determine the most suitable way this might be accomplished."[38] The development in 1964 of a diploma programme in nursing at the Ryerson Institute of Technology, referred to as the "Ryerson Project" was brought about by the Registered Nurses' Association of Ontario in collaboration with the Board of Governors and the Administration of the Ryerson Institute of Technology. The project was approved by the College of Nurses of Ontario, the statutory body administering the Nurses' Act. This assured the graduate of eligibility for registration as a nurse in the province of Ontario.

From the beginning of the project, it was the intention of the Registered Nurses' Association of Ontario to engage in pertinent research. At the present time an intensive research study has been designed to examine the values of the project as a possible solution to the problems confronting nursing education.

In accordance with the Royal Commission on Health Services' recommendation "that there be established in each province a Nursing Education Planning Committee,"[39] the Minister of Public

Health, in Saskatchewan, appointed an ad hoc committee on nursing education in 1965. The report of this committee outlined a proposal for the transfer of the responsibility of nursing education to the Minister of Education, and that a Board of Nursing Education be established by law and that this board be responsible to the Minister of Education. These concepts were accepted and embodied in an amendment to the Department of Education Act and in the Nurses' Education Act, 1966.[40] As an outcome of this report, steps have been taken to phase out the existing hospital schools and to develop two central schools of nursing in Regina and Saskatoon. The first central school of nursing established in the Institute of Applied Arts and Sciences in Saskatoon opened in September 1967. The second school is to be established in Regina and it is hoped that it will be part of a community college programme.[41]

At the present time, programmes similar in concept to the two preceding examples have been established in British Columbia, Alberta, and Quebec. An alternative programme in diploma nursing education emerged in Ontario in 1960 with the development of the Nightingale School of Nursing in Toronto. This school was considered to be a regional school – one which controls the educational programme and utilizes the resources within a geographic area. Its genesis reflected the support of the Board of Governors of the New Mount Sinai Hospital for a school which embraced the same principles of administration inherent in the first Nightingale School of Nursing established by Florence Nightingale in 1860. The cost of constructing the school, erected on land donated by the Board of Governors of the New Mount Sinai Hospital, was borne by the government of Ontario. Its operating costs have continued to be derived from the Ontario Hospital Services Commission.

In the province of Ontario, a marked expansion in recruitment into diploma school programmes was initiated in 1965 by the provincial Department of Health. The proposed plan was based upon an estimated need to double the number of nurses in graduating classes from 2500 to 5000 within a five-year period. Under the expansion programme the following steps were to be taken: the length of the educational program was to be reduced to two years; a third, or internship year in hospital nursing service, would be required during the transitional period from 1965 to 1975; the school would be under the direction of a board; the school would have its own budget controlled by its board; existing schools were to expand physical facilities to accommodate an increased enrolment of students; new regional schools were to be built which would use the clinical resources of several hospitals located in a geographic area where a school had not been previously located or where an existing school would phase into a new identity.[42]

The financing of these expanded nursing education programmes at the diploma level in Ontario, with the exception of the one offered by Ryerson, was the responsibility of the Department of Health. The money for operating expenses was channelled through the Ontario Hospital Services Commission via the per diem rate paid to the hospitals which owned the schools or to designated hospitals in the case of regional schools.

Although the emphasis in this chapter has been on the development of diploma-level nursing education, it should be recalled that the recommended ratio of nurses prepared at the baccalaureate level to nurses prepared at the diploma level should be 1 : 3. This factor must be considered in evaluating the qualitative success of the quantitative expansion evident in a comparison of enrolment figures in Ontario for the years 1965 and 1968 in each type of programme (see Table 1).

A study of enrolment figures raises many questions. What is the ideal level of enrolment? In Ontario in 1968, annual enrolment ranged from 25 to 178 in sixty-three programmes. Eight schools

TABLE 1

| | | 1965 | | 1968 | |
| | | Number of programmes | Number of students | Number of programmes | Number of students |
Type of programme	Length of programme				
University (baccalaureate)	4 years	3	121	7	241
Diploma	2 years	3	138	9	703
	2 years with a third year of nursing service	9	830	43	2817
	3 years	49	2506	11	424
	TOTAL	64	3595	70	4185

SOURCE: College of Nurses of Ontario, "*Admissions to Schools of Nursing,*" (Toronto, 1965–68).

enrolled more than 100 students, twenty-nine enrolled 50 to 100 students, and twenty-six enrolled between 25 and 49 students. Is the best use being made of financial resources? Programmes may have few or many students enrolled, be widespread geographically, or be concentrated. In Toronto there were fifteen diploma programmes with enrolment between 26 and 130 in individual schools in 1968, but whose collective enrolment accounted for approximately one-third of the provincial total. Is it feasible to recruit the necessary administrative and teaching staff for the total number of programmes in the province when their source emanates from the university nursing programmes at the baccalaureate or master's level which in addition must provide leaders in nursing service in hospitals and other health agencies at the provincial, national, and international levels?

In this historical résumé of the development of nursing education at the diploma level, emphasis has been placed on those forces in society which tended to implement the principle of nursing education enunciated by Florence Nightingale; namely, a school of nursing is an educational entity with financial and administrative autonomy. Among the counterforces that attenuated the application of this principle was the influence of "voluntarism" with its dependence upon philanthropy, fees paid by patients, and student services to defray the cost of providing hospital services. This system has undergone and is undergoing critical review as a result of the advent of prepaid hospital insurance plans. These plans are now administered by provincial government departments or commissions. This requires the public through their elected representatives to assess the need for nurses on a much broader basis than the needs of an individual hospital. Dr. Matthew B. Dymond, former Minister of Health in the province of Ontario, reflected this attitude at a conference of directors of Schools of Nursing, when he stated,

The nurse today has to be well educated if she is to fill her proper role in the health programmes. ... Arising out of the continuing dialogue on education, is the question of – "Where should the responsibility for Nursing Education lie? Should it be part of the function of the Department of Education along with "general education"? Should it lie with the Universities? Should it remain where it traditionally has been – as part of the Department of Health?

Good and valid arguments can be put forward to support or reject each and all of these views. ... As in all education, if [nursing education] is to prosper and make its fullest contribution to Society, all of us must approach these questions with open and inquiring minds.[43]

The question remains, in Ontario, as in all of Canada, where should the ultimate responsibility for the administration and financing of diploma programmes in nursing education rest? Surveys, commissions, and studies have all pointed to the inescapable conclusion that nursing education has the right to public support and that it belongs in educational institutions under educational auspices. While the hospital-owned and -controlled school of nursing may have been the best solution in the past to society's search for a supply of nurses, today's diploma programmes are undergoing radical revision as society searches for answers to the following questions:

Can single-discipline schools of nursing, which isolate their students from society's mainstream of students who receive a liberal along with a technical education, prepare nurses to meet the needs of a society that demands a space-age style of nursing?

Is it appropriate that the funds for the current upgrading of single-discipline schools, hospital or regional, should come from the hospital insurance dollar, be administered by a hospital services commission, and be included in the cost of providing a hospital service?

Is the maintenance of residences where students are accommodated without personal costs, a justifiable component in the "costs" of nursing education?

Is an internship year of required nursing service a justifiable component of a programme in nursing education?

At a time when the total framework of education is changing to offer citizens of all ages opportunities consistent with their abilities and aspirations, surely the unequal educational opportunities for nursing students at the diploma level cannot continue to be unrecognized and unresolved. Until a major effort is made by governments, hospitals, health professions and the public to integrate the education of nurses into the mainstream of the country's educational systems, the preparation of today's nurse will be deficient in those liberal and technological components required to meet the future demands that will be made of nursing.

NOTES

1 Donald Creighton, *Dominion of the North* (Toronto, 1947), p. 40.
2 John Murray Gibbon and Mary Matthewson, *Three Centuries of Canadian Nursing* (Toronto, 1947), p. 3.
3 *Ibid.*, p. 2.
4 *Ibid.*, p. 155.
5 Josephine Goldmark, *Nursing and Nursing Education in the United States* (New York, 1923).
6 *Ibid.*, p. 202.
7 George M. Weir, *Survey of Nursing Education in Canada* (Toronto, 1932), p. 9.
8 *Ibid.*, p. 48.
9 *Ibid.*, pp. 466–7.
10 Canadian Nurses' Association, *Proposed Curriculum Guide for Schools of Nursing in Canada* (Montreal, 1936), p. 6.
11 *Ibid.*, p. 15.
12 *Ibid.*
13 Canadian Nurses' Association, "Statement of Policies" (Ottawa, April 1951).
14 *Report of Committee of Canadian Red Cross Society*, Nov. 4, 1946.
15 Arthur R. Lord, *Report of the Evaluation of the Metropolitan School of Nursing* (Ottawa, 1952).
16 *Ibid.*, p. 54.
17 Edith Kathleen Russell, *The Report of a Study in Nursing Education in New Brunswick* (Fredericton, 1956), p. 25.
18 W. Stewart Wallace, *Report of the Experiment in Nursing Education of the Atkinson School of Nursing, Toronto Western Hospital, 1950–1955* (Toronto, 1955), p. 9.
19 *Ibid.*, p. 11.
20 *Ibid.*, p. 9.
21 *Ibid.*, p. 17.
22 Helen K. Mussallem, *Spotlight on Nursing Education* (Ottawa, 1960), p. 2.
23 *Ibid.*, p. 2.
24 *Ibid.*, p. 88.
25 *Ibid.*, p. 89.
26 Katherine E. MacLaggan, "Bill 320 and the Student of Nursing," *Canadian Nurse* LIV (May 1958): 409.
27 *Report of the Royal Commission on Health Services* (Ottawa, 1964), vol. I.
28 Helen K. Mussallem, *Nursing Education in Canada* (Ottawa, 1965), p. 2.
29 *Ibid.*, pp. 137–8.
30 *Report of the Royal Commission on Health Services*, p. 579.
31 *Ibid.*, p. 67.
32 *Ibid.*, p. 585.
33 *Ibid.*, p. 593.
34 Canadian Nurses' Association, "Submission to the Royal Commission on Health Services," March 1962, p. 31.
35 School of Nursing, University of Toronto, "Brief to the Royal Commission on Health Services," May 1962, p. 12.
36 *Ibid.*, p. 13.

37 Registered Nurses' Association of Ontario, "Submission to the Royal Commission on Health Services," May 1962, p. iii.
38 *Ibid.*
39 *Report of the Royal Commission on Health Services*, p. 67.
40 *Report of the Ad Hoc Committee on Nursing Education, Province of Saskatchewan* (Regina, 1966).
41 Linda Long, "Tomorrow's Nursing Education in Saskatchewan," *The Canadian Nurse* LXIII (April 1967): 33.
42 "Proposals for the Future Pattern of Nursing Education in Ontario; A Summary of Papers Presented at a Series of Nursing Education Conferences" (June 1965).
43 Matthew B. Dymond, "The Winds of Change," Address to the Conference of Directors of Schools of Nursing, Toronto, February 1968, p. 13.

7
The emergence of the nursing assistant

MARJORIE G. RUSSELL

Dr. Kathleen Russell made the comment that "it is the official approval of the Auxiliary that is new, not the worker."[1] Practical
nurses, many without any formal training, have been used as long
as one can remember. These women have given nursing care in the
home; but before the advent of the course for nursing assistants,
nursing in the hospitals was provided entirely by registered and
student nurses. Registered nurses were generally in administrative,
supervisory, and teaching positions, whereas the greater part of
bedside care was given by students. Some assistance was provided
for the nurse by attendants, aides, and orderlies; these were trained
for particular duties by the hospital that employed them. Attendants,
both male and female, were used largely in institutions caring for
the mentally ill, and made up a large proportion of the staff in those
departments that provided custodial care. A small number of orderlies and ward aides were employed by most general hospitals.
Their duties included simple measures which provided for the comfort of the patient, such as making beds, carrying trays, and caring
for equipment. For example, the Hospital for Sick Children in Toronto trained a small number of girls as nursery aides to assist in the
Infant Department with bathing and feeding babies and looking
after linen and other supplies. During the war, orderlies and sick
berth attendants were given short courses in elementary nursing,
and many of these men are now orderlies in the hospitals for Veterans Affairs.

In the early years of the Second World War, the Canadian Nurses'
Association saw that something must be done to meet the need for
more adequate nursing throughout the country; and the necessity of

establishing schools for nursing assistants in all provinces was foreseen. As an important function of the Association is to foster high standards of nursing practice, it was considered that licensing and control of the auxiliary was an urgent matter; and a recommendation was made to the provinces that immediate steps be taken to effect suitable legislation for the nursing assistant. A syllabus for the course, to be used as a guide by provincial nursing associations, was developed by the Canadian Nurses' Association, and recommendations were made regarding the functions, qualifications, and preparation of the "nursing assistant" which was the title suggested by the Association for this group. These recommendations called for the maintenance of standards of care through the guidance, support, and supervision of the nursing assistant by provincial nursing associations. This was the spearhead, so to speak, of the nursing-assistant programme in Canada. The provinces responded to the need. The guidelines enunciated by the Canadian Nurses' Association were approved, and schools were established in each province.

Ontario, which was the first province to secure legislation for the nursing assistant, will serve as an illustration of the origin and development of this programme.

Discussion about the advisability of providing a course of training for practical nurses in Ontario first took place in 1939. Under the Nursing Act, nursing education was the responsibility of the Department of Health. A Council of Nurse Education advised the minister on matters affecting standards, and regulations were administered by the Nursing Branch of the department.

At this time there were several small hospitals in the province whose schools of nursing did not meet the minimum requirements under the regulations and whose graduates could not be registered under the Nursing Act. In a committee composed of the Council of Nurse Education and members of the Registered Nurses' Association of Ontario, the question was raised as to whether the graduates of these schools should be considered as part of the group of practical nurses now employed in homes. This group was made up of an undetermined number of women who had obtained their knowledge of nursing either through experience or in schools in the community that gave varying amounts of training and operated under private auspices not subject to any standard or control. One such school had no regular order of procedure; a student could enter at any time, and could be given the diploma of the school without having to subject herself to any examination of her knowledge. Yet these schools were the only means of supplying a sense of satisfaction and an income to a large number of women whose desire was to nurse, but whose education fell short of the minimum standards for entry to an approved school of nursing. Though many practical nurses performed a valuable service in the community, the methods used by the schools of practical nursing gave cause for concern within the nursing profession in regard to the welfare of the public, who were generally unaware of the capabilities of the practical nurse.

Since practical nurses worked in homes, under medical direction, the committee decided at this time to obtain a sampling of opinion from medical practitioners as to the safety and effectiveness of their work. Accordingly, the medical associations of two counties in the province were approached for information. A survey was made, and the opinions of the doctors consulted pointed to the need of better training for the practical nurse as well as registration for her. It was felt by these doctors that this would benefit both the patient and the doctor by providing a stated level of competence that might be expected from the practical nurse. She in turn would benefit from a course that would be organized to teach her the necessary skills for her work, and she would receive a recognized status in the community.

In January 1940, a tentative plan was drawn up for the training of the practical nurse. This plan included the establishment of a central school which would have an affiliation with a group of hospitals, preferably hospitals without nursing schools, where the students could obtain supervised practical experience. It was proposed that the training would start with four months in the central school, where the student would be taught the basic nursing skills she would be expected to use; and that this would be followed by experience with children and adults in the affiliated hospitals. The course would conclude with a final period at the school. During this time some supervised practice in homes could be given. Licensing of the graduate of this school was also seen as necessary.

Meanwhile, a shortage of nurses was beginning to develop in hospitals throughout the province. During the late 1930s a gradual change had taken place in the staffing of hospitals. An increasing number of registered nurses were being employed for general staff duties. In addition to this, nurses were taking advantage of offers to registered nurses for general ward duty in hospitals in the United States. The Second World War had begun, and many nurses were leaving hospitals to join the armed services. Shortages were felt particularly in the larger centres where hospital units were being set up for both home and overseas service. In these centres a substantial number of nurses and doctors were recruited from a few hospitals.

How much of the shortage was due to a lack of nurses and how much to the use or misuse of a nurse's time is a matter of conjecture. Traditionally, nurses have carried out numerous duties which, while necessary to the well-being and comfort of the patient, belong in the category of housekeeping, dietary, clerical, and other services, and this has reduced the amount of nursing care that could be given. The nurse in a hospital is available twenty-four hours a day, and this availability places her in a position where she has been required to assume some of the responsibilities of other disciplines and departments. Most departments in the hospital are open only for the length of the normal working day. This means that during the hours between the closing and reopening of these departments the nurse has been expected in many instances to extend her role to include that of the administrator, the pharmacist, the dietitian, and others. The removal of such extra responsibilities from nurses could have made a considerable amount of additional nursing care available.

Demands for nursing services continued to grow, and it became a matter of some urgency to find a way of meeting these demands. Since it was impossible to get enough registered nurses, some other means of assistance would have to be found. There were patients in hospitals who were convalescing, and some with chronic illnesses, whose nursing needs were simple in nature. It was recognized that some of their care could be safely delegated to an auxiliary worker if this person were given a suitable course of training and worked under the direction of a registered nurse. Preparing a course of training, and finding financial assistance for it, would be only the beginning. If such a programme was to be successful there were other important factors to consider. If a new assistant to the nurse was to be brought into the hospital, the hospital staff would require an understanding of her training, capabilities, and limitations. The safety and protection of the patient must be a major concern of all those involved in the training and use of this assistant, and it would be important to see that she had the proper direction and supervision.

By the spring of 1941 the Registered Nurses' Association of Ontario had prepared an outline for a course of training. It was decided that this should be used as a demonstration to determine the feasibility of training an auxiliary group, under approved educational principles, to assist the nurse in the hospital and to provide a well-trained person for nursing care in homes. The Association was prepared to finance such a course for the duration of the demonstration. Approval was secured from the Council of Nurse Education of the Ontario Department of Health for the demonstration to be carried out, and the first students were admitted to classes in September of the same year. The course was conducted with the co-operation of the Nursing Registry in London, and eight classes were admitted before it was discontinued in 1945. The purpose of the training was to prepare an auxiliary worker (1) to nurse the convalescent, chronically ill, and medical and surgical patient where simple nursing skill is required, and (2) to work in conjunction with a registered nurse where skilled nursing care is required. It was emphasized that the graduate from this course was trained to supplement the nurse, and that she should work under the direction of a nurse in the hospital.

The length of the course was set at six months, and completion of the grade 8 certificate in Ontario was determined as the standard for admission. For the first three and a half months students were to attend a central school and follow this with supervised experience in hospitals caring for convalescent and chronically ill children and adults. It was planned that some experience in homes was to follow under the direction of the Victorian Order of Nurses.

With the exception of a small tuition fee, the Registered Nurses' Association paid for all expenses incurred during the course. These expenses were kept to a minimum through the co-operation and help of the agencies that agreed to participate in the training. Classrooms, supervised practice, and medical services were provided for the students without charge.

When the course was terminated, eight classes had been admitted and 106 students graduated. As there was no provision for licensing of this assistant at that time, the graduates were required to identify themselves with a community nursing registry.

When the graduates of this course were employed in hospitals, it soon became evident that they were filling a need; and the Registered Nurses' Association recommended to the provincial government that schools for nursing assistants be established independently of hospitals in centres large enough to provide practice for the students in hospitals and homes in the community.

At the end of the war, when members of the armed forces were released from service, the federal government recognized the need to help these veterans return to civilian life, and government funds were made available for this purpose. Under this arrangement, plans were made through the Departments of Veterans Affairs, the national and provincial Nursing Associations, and the departments of Health and Education in the provinces, to organize courses for the training of practical nurses. In Ontario, this programme was conducted during the year 1946, and was terminated at the end of the year when this segment of the population was served. The total number of auxiliaries prepared in these courses was relatively small.

During this year, the Department of Health in Ontario conducted a survey to find out how many people were helping to give nursing care, and what methods were being used to teach them. The survey revealed that over four hundred were receiving some type of training to assist with nursing duties. Much of the instruction was given on the job and consisted of a few hours of nursing demonstrations weekly. In other cases, courses were given which covered periods of from eighteen months to three years. The findings of this survey supported the need for a suitable programme of training for auxiliaries in nursing, and convinced the provincial authorities that it was a matter of urgency to establish a course for nursing assistants. In 1947 training centres opened in Toronto and Kingston under the joint sponsorship of the departments of Health and Education of the province. The course followed the recommendations of the Canadian Nurses' Association and was approved by the Registered Nurses' Association of Ontario. A monthly allowance was given to each student to assist with maintenance during the course. The director of the nursing branch stated in her report of that year that "the success of the training course for nursing assistants will be judged by the standards of service given, and will depend on guidance given by all nurses in the province."[2] She emphasized that the function of the nursing assistant is to supplement, not to replace, the professional nurse.

It was impossible to tell what the response to the course would be; but with the numbers of practical nurses working in the community it was evident that there was much interest in nursing. The sponsors thought that recruitment might be influenced by the fact that the course was designed with particular reference to maintaining student status for the recruit, and that when she graduated she would have an assured place in the community, with expectation of employment in a hospital. Events proved the popularity of the course with both students and employers, and subsequently other training centres were opened.

In the same year an amendment to the Nurses' Act was made. This included regulations for setting up training centres, the qualifications of entry, the content and length of the course, and the licensing of the graduates. The regulations also made provision that a hospital able to meet the qualifications could seek approval as a training centre; and a number of hospitals have been given authority for this. With this legislation, steps were taken to recognize those who had formerly been trained under approved auspices, and the graduates of the courses sponsored by the Registered Nurses' Association and those of the Canadian Vocational Training Schools were registered by waiver.

Eventually, training for nursing assistants was brought into the Ontario vocational school system. In 1953 the Council of Nurse Education recommended to the Minister of Health that the departments of Health and Education of the province explore the possibility of using the facilities of vocational schools to teach courses for nursing assistants. Four years later a pilot project, made possible by means of a federal health grant, was begun at the H. B. Beal Technological and Commercial High School in London. This course was planned to provide a programme during the third and fourth years of secondary school, which would divide its curriculum equally between academic and nursing subjects, the latter to include suitable practice in hospitals.

This project was seen as a means of bringing the nursing assistant programme within the general educational system of the province and at the same time keeping a number of students in school who would otherwise drop out. The choice of this course would give them their secondary school graduation diploma and at the same time make available to them a vocational training that would provide them with an occupation on graduation. Until this time the only vocational courses open to girls had been in home economics and commercial subjects. Of the original class of eleven graduates, six were employed as nursing assistants and five entered a school of nursing. Ten other vocational schools have since offered the same programme. In 1968, 368 students were enrolled in the nursing assistant courses. Male students have been enrolled since the beginning of these programmes, but their numbers have been small so far.

In the same year that the first vocational school course was offered, the Toronto Training Centre instituted an evening course for nursing assistants. This programme consists of an eight-month period during which the students attend evening classes. It is followed by four months of clinical practice, after which students become eligible for examination. In 1968 there were 55 centres in the province for teaching nursing assistants. These centres admitted 2253 students. To date there appears to be no lack of applicants for this course in Ontario.

When the training of nursing assistants was first introduced in Canada, it was seen as a means of providing additional nursing care in hospitals during the war years. But when the war was over and nurses returned from overseas, there still remained a shortage of nursing service. Various factors contributed to this. Hospitals were enlarging their facilities, and new hospitals were being built. The demand for health services in the community was increasing. Advances in medical science were introducing new patterns in the treatment and care of patients. These changes were progressing at an ever-increasing rate, and it appeared that in the foreseeable future there would be a need to continue with the nursing assistant programmes.

Canada has not been alone in using the nursing assistant. A move toward the use of auxiliary nursing personnel had taken place in many countries. In 1950 the World Health Organization made a study of the need to provide adequate nursing services throughout the world, and the Expert Committee on Nursing concluded that in order to do this, three approaches would be necessary. These were: (1) securing candidates for training of all types, (2) promotion of the most effective use of various types of nursing personnel, and (3) provision of educational facilities and programmes for all types of nurses needed. The report of this committee stated that "many nursing activities formerly performed by nurses can be safely entrusted to workers with less comprehensive training."[3] It also considered "the employment of auxiliary nursing personnel an essential factor in the provision of nursing services in homes and in hospitals, general and special, including tuberculosis sanatoriums, mental hospitals, and institutions for chronic patients."[4] A later report of this organization stated that there is "considerable evidence that there is an important and continuing place for the auxiliary workers in public health to perform the many duties which require less independent judgement than is expected of professional nurses."[5]

From the beginning, the Canadian Nurses' Association has been vitally concerned with the preparation and use of the nursing assistant. In its advisory capacity the Association has felt a responsibility to establish a guide to assist the provincial nursing associations in directing the programmes wisely and committees of the Association have continued to study the training and use of the nursing assistant in providing nursing service. By 1950 several schools had been opened in the provinces, and the Association decided that the time was ripe for a thorough study of the whole problem of the role of auxiliary workers in the present-day programme of providing nursing service to the public. A committee was appointed to review the programmes and make recommendations. From the information available it was decided that there was a need to continue the training of the nursing assistant if all parts of the country were to be served, but that there should be some standardization of this training. To assist with this, suggestions were made as follows:

1 There should be an advisory committee to the school.
2 The school should be separate from a hospital, with clinical experience available for the student.
3 The ratio of teachers to students should be 1 to 20 and the teacher should have a thorough understanding of the role of the nursing assistant.
4 The age for admission should be between 18 and 40 years.
5 The length of the course should not exceed nine months.
6 The curriculum should follow that prepared by the Canadian Nurses' Association.
7 The student should have a distinctive uniform with identification.
8 Male students should be admitted to the course.

There was one addition to the curriculum. Because patients, including children, were taught to give themselves insulin injections, it was decided that nursing assistants should also be taught this technique for use in homes.

One point of great importance was interpretation of the role of the nursing assistant to both the medical and nursing professions. The report of the committee went on to say, "It has been established that the nursing assistant has an important place in the total health pro- gramme. If she is to be used to best advantage it is essential that there should exist a thorough understanding of her role."[6]

The number of nursing assistant programmes grew steadily, until by 1960 there were forty-three throughout Canada with an enrol- ment of 2200 students. These courses varied in length from nine to eighteen months. In some cases schools were being asked to teach nursing procedures that had not been approved as coming within the scope of the nursing assistant. The Canadian Nurses' Association felt that if a trend toward increasing the teaching – and thereby per- mitting the nursing assistant to increase her role – were to continue, the distinction between what the nurse was responsible for and what the nursing assistant was doing would become increasingly blurred; the result would be confusion and difficulty in maintaining satisfac- tory standards of care. A study of nursing education and service in Canada was being made at this time, and the Canadian Nurses' As- sociation recommended that the curriculum for nursing assistant courses should not be changed until future policy could be deter- mined.

The more or less rapid supply of nursing assistants posed many problems for agencies and professional staff. The speed with which she appeared on the scene once the training programmes got under way, and the relatively limited time available to prepare those who would be working with her to understand her capabilities and limita- tions, has made it difficult to avoid some misuse and confusion. A good deal of credit must be given to those who have been able to direct the nursing assistant so that she is using her training without either a waste of her skills or an overstepping of her responsibilities.

From her preparation it could be assumed that convalescent patients and many with chronic disabilities could be competently cared for by the nursing assistant with a minimum of supervision. But although it is true that for many of these patients the nursing care that is required is relatively simple, there are possibly as many who need the support and rehabilitative nursing that should be given by a registered nurse. If these patients are to get this kind of care it would be necessary to bring the new assistant into a plan where the care of the patient is divided between the nurse and the assistant, according to the patient's need and how much of this the assistant is capable of giving.

One attempt to bring the nursing assistant into a plan of care has been the so-called team approach, initiated in the United States. The Committee on the Function of Nursing saw this approach as placing "its major reliance on the performance of the total nursing mission by a group of nurses in which the essential element is a supervisory relationship between the registered or professional nurse and the practical nurse."[7] This method recognized that individuals with various levels of education and skills could be used more effectively as a team to care for a group of patients than in separate assignments according to the kind of patient to be cared for. If appropriately carried out, it also reduces the number of nursing personnel who contribute to the patient's care, and provides for a continuity of this care, with more satisfaction for the patient and for the worker. This approach places on a registered nurse the responsibility for planning the care for a group of patients and determining how and by whom the care is to be given, calling for a high degree of knowledge and skill.

The original object in preparing a nursing assistant was to provide help for the hospitals; and approximately 95 per cent of these assistants are working in hospitals. A number have found employment with community health agencies, and this has taken them into homes, schools, and clinics. There are also a few in industry. In these situations the nursing assistant works under the direction of the public health nurse.

An example of the use of the nursing assistant in one of these agencies may be seen in the work of the Victorian Order of Nurses. Because of a marked increase in the number of patients with chronic illness, the Order found it necessary to expand its service. It was not possible to obtain enough nurses to meet this demand, so in 1947 an experiment was carried out by the Victorian Order in Toronto to find out how nursing assistants could be used in a programme of home care. This experiment was based on the hypothesis that "patients with chronic illness require care of the highest quality; and at the same time the special skills and knowledge of the public health nurse are being dissipated if the preponderance of her service is devoted to patients with chronic illnesses."[8] A plan was drawn up, in which the nursing assistant would give care under the close supervision of the nurse to selected patients whose nursing needs were stabilized. The plan was carefully interpreted to doctors, patients, and the public; and the nursing assistant was introduced to home care. It was found that the care the nursing assistant gave under this team relationship was very satisfactory, which was an encouraging factor in the employment of more nursing assistants. The views of the Order are shown in the statement: "In concluding its experiment the Toronto Branch of the Victorian Order of Nurses feels that the use of the certified nursing assistant has been amply demonstrated and now considers this worker as an essential member of its nursing team."[9]

Since the establishment of the schools for nursing assistants, all provinces, except Quebec and Newfoundland, provide recognition for the graduates through legislation. In most of the provinces, certification or registration is provided for, through either the provincial Departments of Health or the Registered Nurses' Associations. In Nova Scotia, the Board of Registration of Nursing Assistants is the licensing body; in Ontario, the College of Nurses.

Because the development of the nursing assistant programme in Ontario has been used as an example, a brief résumé of the legislation for nursing assistants in this province is included here. When the Registered Nurses' Association of Ontario was studying the need for a programme for training nursing assistants in 1940, licensing and control of this assistant was seen as mandatory. As the province administered the Nurses' Act at that time, the Association adopted a resolution asking the Department of Health to enact legislation that would provide for licensing and approval of courses of training for nursing assistants.

With the advent of the course, in which the Departments of Health and Education were involved, the Nurses' Act was amended. In March 1947 regulations were made under this Act, which made provision for the training and registration of the nursing assistant. This legislation established the title, Certified Nursing Assistant. Registration was open to all those who had successfully completed the demonstration courses during 1941–45, and to former members of the armed services who had completed the course for practical nurses under the Canadian government vocational training scheme in Ontario.

When the first nursing legislation was established in Ontario, the control of nursing education and minimum standards came under the jurisdiction of the Department of Health. In the amended Act no change was made in this; but when the Nurses Registration Act of 1951 gave the Registered Nurses' Association authority to set standards and control the education and registration of nurses, control of the nursing assistant was retained by the Department of Health. With the Nurses' Act 1961–62, which established the College of Nurses of Ontario as the governing body of the nursing profession, provision for governing nursing assistants was included.

Regulations under this Act govern the standards for training centres, the content and length of the course, and the requirements for admission to training; and provide for the inspection of these centres. Provision is also made for the examination of graduates from Ontario schools, the examination or registration of nursing assistants from other provinces, and the renewal, suspension, or cancellation of registration.

Some flexibility has been introduced into the standards of admission to register. In 1955 regulations under the Nursing Act were waived in order to register by examination former graduates of courses conducted in public general hospitals whose programmes did not meet the requirements for nurse registration. A waiver was introduced again in 1961 which made provision for any person who had clinical and theoretical training in nursing in Ontario, who had been employed in a public general hospital for a minimum of five years, performing the same duties as a nursing assistant, and who was recommended by the employer. More recently, a new regulation of the College makes provision for the Council of the College to register, at its discretion, any person who has successfully completed a course for aides and attendants, which has been conducted by a hospital within the meaning of the Mental Hospitals Act – from 1952 until July 1969. This waiver will be in effect until June 1970.

Graduates of the schools are known in the different provinces as: registered or certified nursing assistants, certified nursing aides, and licensed practical nurses.

The programmes for the courses are based on the outline recommended by the Canadian Nurses' Association. There are variations in entrance requirements, length of courses, age, and emoluments.

In two provinces the educational qualification for entry to the course is grade 9; in six provinces it is grade 10. Ontario has the shortest course, thirty-five weeks; Alberta follows with forty weeks. In the other provinces, courses are of either ten or twelve months' duration, except for Quebec's, which is eighteen months. Six of these eighteen months are regarded as an internship.

The minimum age for entry to the schools is usually seventeen years, but three provinces require the applicant to have passed her eighteenth birthday. The maximum age varies from forty years up. A tuition fee of $60.00 is required in British Columbia. In Nova Scotia one school, that of the Department of Veterans Affairs, requires a $40.00 fee. Most other programmes have no tuition fees, and some provinces provide weekly or monthly allowances for students, which vary. Students in Alberta are given $3.00 per day, whereas those in Nova Scotia receive $80.00 per month. In some cases room and board is provided.

Associations of nursing assistants have been formed in most provinces, but as yet there is no national association. In all provinces except British Columbia liaison is maintained between the Registered Nurses' Association and the Association of Nursing Assistants. This is done through representation on the advisory council or executive committees of the Association of Nursing Assistants, by the Registered Nurses' Association in the province.

While it is recognized that the introduction of the nursing assistant programme has been a realistic approach to the demand for nursing service, there have been a number of problems in making the best use of the graduate. In many situations the extent of her training has been well understood and good use has been made of her contribution. In these situations her functions are well defined; she is well directed and supervised and gives quality care. But there are also situations in which she has been asked to function beyond the level of her knowledge, with or without being given additional teaching. This may be due to a lack of knowledge of her training, or to an insufficient number of registered nurses in the hospital; but it can only result in inadequate care for the patient. There are, too, situations in which full recognition is not given to what she is trained to do, and many of the duties that are assigned to her should properly be the responsibility of the housekeeping or some other department. Both of these practices present a questionable use of the nursing assistant.

Problems in the use of the nursing assistant have emerged in other countries that have been struggling to provide much-needed additional nursing service. In 1960 a report of the International Labour Organization on the employment and conditions of the work of nurses, made the comment that "in many cases the employment and utilization of auxiliary personnel has been an improvised response to immediate needs; they have not been the outgrowth of a concerted plan of work allocation and organization."[10] This publication also says, "A basic problem of effective utilization of existing personnel is linked with the definition of nursing functions. What are the proper duties of professional nurses? What functions can be performed effectively by auxiliary nursing staff? What can be done to conserve nursing energies for the performance of professional functions?"[11]

The number of nursing assistants in Canada has been growing rapidly. There are now over 30,000 registered or licensed nursing assistants in Canada and there appears to be no shortage of applicants for these courses.

It has been pointed out that "of all the categories of workers in the health occupations prepared through educational programmes, none has increased more rapidly over the past 20 years than the nursing assistant ... the numbers graduating from schools for nursing assistants have increased dramatically in comparison with graduates from basic nursing programmes. If the present trend continues new nursing assistant graduates could eventually outnumber new graduates from professional schools of nursing."[12]

In all provinces many of the applicants to nursing assistant courses have academic qualifications in excess of the minimum (grade 9 or 10) and these numbers appear to be increasing yearly. During 1968, in Ontario 56.4 per cent had qualifications above the minimum. Of these, 38.9 per cent were eligible to enter a diploma course in nursing.

What is the future of the nursing assistant? The registered nurse in the hospital has gradually been forced to relinquish much of the direct nursing care she has formerly given. Many nurses who find their greatest satisfaction in giving personal care to the patient now find that it is not possible for them to devote as much time as they would like to all the patients who need care. During the last twenty years changes have been brought about which have added to the nurse's responsibilities. She is now using complicated therapeutic equipment; she is being asked to assume an increasing number of tasks formerly performed by doctors; more of her time must be spent in teaching patients and supervising the work of others. All of these have contributed to the fact that a great deal of bedside nursing care is being given by the nursing assistant.

Many nursing assistants are dissatisfied with their lack of opportunity for advancement. They are anxious to extend their knowledge and improve their skills. They feel the need for refresher courses and would like an opportunity to take post-basic courses such as in psychiatric nursing.

The Canadian Nurses' Association has expressed the opinion that in order to resolve some of the difficulties that are emerging with regard to the training and use of the nursing assistant an eventual merging of graduates of diploma schools of nursing and nursing assistants is desirable. In its brief to the Royal Commission on Health Services, the Association stated:

The Association is concerned about the proliferation of workers in nursing. Too often – at least to the patient – the patient belongs to no one and no one belongs to the patient. Besides the interference of nurse-patient relationship it gives rise to overlapping and duplication of activities and results in the fragmentation of patient care.

The performance by nursing assistants of nursing functions beyond the worker's preparation and often without competent supervision, may jeopardize the quality of care given and the safety and well being of patients.

The Canadian Nurses' Association therefore believes that nursing service can best be met through the consolidation of current categories of nursing personnel into fewer, possibly two groups which can be differentiated on the basis of function and education.[13]

It is considered that these two categories would include graduates from university and diploma schools of nursing, whereas the courses for nursing assistants would be gradually discontinued. As we have already seen, a large number of present nursing assistant students would qualify for entry to a diploma school leading to registration as a nurse. At the general meeting of the Canadian Nurses' Association in 1968, approval was given to a recommendation of the Committee on Nursing Education that, "all programmes which prepare practitioners, who, upon graduation, are not eligible for licensure as registered nurses be gradually phased out."[14] Some nurses, however, take the position that there is a continuing need for the nursing assistant. They believe that there are many patients in hospitals and homes who do not require bedside care to be given by a registered nurse but can be well and safely cared for by the nursing assistant where a nurse assumes the responsibility for assessment of the patient's needs and directs and supervises the care. This position can be strengthened from an economic standpoint. Is it reasonable to have a registered nurse giving care to all patients if someone with a lesser education can share in giving this care? Should the patient be asked to pay for nursing service he may not require? Should health agencies now satisfactorily employing nursing assistants employ registered nurses instead? These are some of the questions that have been asked.

In its report the Royal Commission on Health Services has said: "Much of the work of the nursing team is to-day performed by the nursing assistant, who in most cases receives a limited formal course that varies from school to school from 10 to 18 months' duration. We foresee a continuation of this category of nursing service. We believe that in view of the reduction of the training of the diploma nurse to two years, the formal training period of the nursing assistant must be shortened. Ultimately perhaps, many will be trained on the job. ... we expect that since a large proportion of those now entering the nursing assistant programme have an educational standard above the required minimum for this programme, many of these girls would consider a career as a diploma nurse as a preferred alternative, particularly when the course is shortened to two years."[15]

What is the future of the nursing assistant in other countries? The World Health Organization's Expert Committee on Nursing said in its report of 1966 that, "there appears to be an unfortunate tendency to underestimate the potential contribution of the auxiliary workers and to regard their work as something the nurse could do better if only she had the time. It seems clear that both the quality and quantity of patient care can be improved by the utilization of a combination of nursing personnel of different categories provided that certain principles are followed. This is based on the philosophy that the individual patient and his problems are the central focus and that nursing functions appropriate to "care" in a given situation can be appropriately distributed among nursing personnel with varying kinds of preparation to the best advantage of the patient."[16]

Will there continue to be someone who will assist the nurse – for some time at least? If so, could one answer to the present dilemma lie in a concerted effort to define more precisely the role of the nursing assistant, and to make better use of her training; to induce the large percentage of those students entering schools for nursing assistants who have suitable qualifications to take the two-year diploma course in nursing; and to retain the formal training programmes for nursing assistants, and bring them to a level which would help to avoid overlapping of function?

Perhaps the key to the place of the nursing assistant in the future is in this statement of the International Council of Nurses: "Any constructive solution must be based on a controlled study of resources and needs of a country, as these present themselves not only to-day, but as they are projected for the future."[17]

NOTES

1 Kathleen E. Russell, *The Report of a Study of Nursing Education in New Brunswick* (Fredericton, 1956), p. 26.
2 Edith R. Dick, *Report of the Nursing Branch*, Ontario Department of Health, R.N.A.O. *News Bulletin* (September 1947), p. 16.
3 The Expert Committee on Nursing, *Report of the First Session*, World Health Organization, Geneva, 1950, p. 8.
4 *Ibid.*, p. 18.
5 The Expert Committee on Nursing, *Report of the Fourth Session*, World Health Organization, Geneva, 1959, p. 27.
6 "Report of the special Committee to Study Auxiliary Nursing Personnel," *Canadian Nurse* (1951): 585.
7 The Committee on the Function of Nursing, *A Programme for the Nursing Profession* (New York, 1948), p. 38.
8 May L. Palk, "The Role of the Nursing Assistant in the V.O.N., Toronto Branch," *Canadian Nurse* (October 1954): 807.
9 *Ibid.*
10 International Labour Organization, *The Employment and Condition of the Work of Nurses* (Geneva, 1960), p. 10.
11 *Ibid.*, p. 44.
12 Helen K. Mussallem, "No Lack of Nurses but a Shortage of Nursing," *Canadian Nurse* (August 1967).
13 Canadian Nurses' Association, "Brief to the Royal Commission on Health Services," 1962.
14 "Identity and Destiny in Saskatoon," *Canadian Nurse* (August 1968), 33.
15 *Report of the Royal Commission on Health Services*, vol. 1 (Ottawa, 1964), pp. 584–5.
16 *The Expert Committee on Nursing*, World Health Organization Technical Report, Series 347 (Geneva, 1966), p. 14.
17 *International Nursing Review* (July 1961), p. 68.

8
An administrator's view of nursing education

J. D. WALLACE

The quality of Nursing in the present and future can hardly be expected
to reach a higher level than the vision and leadership of those who direct
nursing education. It is a startling revelation to see how far Nursing has
yet to go before attaining the ideals set forth so succinctly and courage-
ously by Florence Nightingale in her "Notes on Nursing" published in
1859.

Amy Frances Brown, Ph.D.*

People who have not studied the simple "Notes on Nursing" written
by Florence Nightingale and have not contemplated her life of devotion and dedication to the sick may take exception to the comments
made by nurse-educator and consultant, Amy Frances Brown. They
could well point with pride to the progress in patient-care techniques
developed during the past two decades. They could quite properly
indicate that since the turn of the century, nursing education has
developed from a pure in-hospital apprenticeship programme into a
broad educational experience provided at various levels in universities, community colleges, and hospital diploma schools. The progress that has been made during this time, and particularly during
the past two decades, has been outstanding in both education and
service fields. Unfortunately, this does not alter the truth contained
in the quotation. To date, we have not satisfied the simplest and
most important ideal of Florence Nightingale – the requirement that
the needs of the patient as a complete individual take precedence
over the system.

* Modern Concepts of Hospital Administration (Owen: W. B. Saunders,
  1962).

The greatest deterrent to change is tradition. The two oldest health professions – medicine and nursing – are steeped in tradition. If it were possible to correctly identify changes as either good or bad – and if tradition could be programmed to resist only the bad ones – progress toward the ideal would be accelerated. Unfortunately, we are not yet sophisticated enough to have selective tradition. As a result, modern technology has outstripped the ability of the health professions to use it in the care of patients. We are using pre-industrial-revolution, cottage-industry systems in an age of advanced technology. The needs of the patient have yet to attain priority over the system and Florence Nightingale's ideals have not been realized.

In her day, she took issue with the rigid military system under which she had to do the best she could for sick and wounded soldiers. The history of nursing before her time had gained strong traditional roots in the total dedication to service of the sisters in religious orders. From the period of military traditionalization nursing emerged into the "handmaiden to the physician" era that ingrained rigid codes and methodologies even more deeply. Nursing was just beginning to develop an organizational and educational identity of its own when we entered the present era of professional hospital administration. Frequently heard comments would lead one to believe that many practitioners and educators in nursing are still trying to find a reasonable way around this new obstacle to their goal.

Faye G. Abdillah, in "Patient Centred Approaches to Nursing" states that the bulk of the nation's actively practising nurses are the products of an educational system in nursing that has been centred on procedure and diagnosis and geared to the service needs of hospitals rather than to the needs of patients. This statement is strongly contested by the advocates of hospital-based diploma schools of nursing, and there are many. They point out that this may have been true many years ago, but that the academic portion of the diploma school curriculum has now been enriched to the degree that there is very little return in service from students. In most modern schools, this is a fact that cannot be disputed. The disease-centred approach to nursing education is disappearing. The rigid empirical approach is giving way to a more scientific and patient-centred one. There is still hope that the patient of the future may be looked upon by the health team as something more than an interesting collection of organs and diseases.

The major factor that has delayed the development of a co-ordinated patient-centred approach to nursing education has been the difficulty in establishing a clear-cut body of science that nursing can call its own. The emergence of the clinical specialist in recent years indicates that this is now being accomplished. These are nurses with a primary interest in clinical nursing who receive education at the postgraduate level in various specialties. Thus, nurses who are dedicated to the direct care of patients are provided, for the first time, with the opportunity to advance on the basis of their clinical ability. Prior to this development, the only way open for progress in a hospital setting was through administrative or teaching channels.

One might well wonder why the development of a clear-cut body of science in the clinical nursing field has been so long delayed. Now that one is beginning to emerge, it is interesting to speculate on how far it will be allowed to progress. Will it be supported and nurtured by those who have the determination and vision required to make it flourish or will the traditional patterns of practice of doctors, nurses, and administrators allow it to die on the vine? To reach a logical prediction, one must study the patterns of the past, the facts of the present, and the projected systems for delivering health care in the future. On this basis, we can perhaps predict specific roles for nursing service and nursing education in the future.

Nursing developed initially as a trade whose primary purpose was to provide cheap, if dedicated, labour to the infection-ridden hospitals of the early nineteenth century. Apprentices learned by the repetitious process of observing, helping, and, finally, doing. The work was arduous and unrewarding and was therefore even less attractive than the long hours and poor financial rewards offered to young women in the industries of the day. Because of the complete lack of infection control, many nurses succumbed to the diseases of the patients for whom they were caring. As a result, there was little time for a true learning experience and the educational programme consisted primarily of repetitive doing on a trial and error basis. One might well wonder if the term "practice" came into its own during that era.

The hospitals of the first half of the nineteenth century were looked upon by most of society as pest houses to which one went only for the purpose of dying. They were staffed by a few trained doctors and nurses and considerable numbers of completely untrained and unqualified personnel. What little administration there was became the responsibility of the senior sister or nurse and it was up to her to find the funds required for the maintenance of at least a minimal level of service. For the most part, they were charitable institutions operated by religious organizations. Later in the century, municipal governments began to provide some financial assistance but only in rare instances was this adequate to provide acceptable levels of care. As a result, hospitals were for the poor and needy. More affluent citizens preferred to die in the comfort of their own homes.

It was not until 1859, when Florence Nightingale made her views on the educational process known, that the pattern began to change and an organized preceptor system emerged. Graduates and students were paired on a one-to-one basis thus enhancing the "observing" and "helping" features of the apprenticeship programme and eventually improving the quality of the "doing."

At about the same time, the arts of medicine and nursing began to move cautiously into the era of asepsis. It had become obvious that the previous state of affairs could not be allowed to continue if progress in health care was to be made. Detailed studies of hospital care and of educational programmes for doctors and nurses were carried out. The reports that were made to professional and public bodies resulted in dramatic changes in the organization and management of hospitals.

Very few specific drugs had been developed by that time and the treatment of disease was primarily symptomatic. The laying on of hands and a sympathetic approach were still the basic features of the diagnostic and treatment armamentorium, but at least the hands were now aseptic. As a result, mortality and morbidity rates began to improve and hospitals became accepted by the public as good places in which to receive treatment.

Organized nursing originated in North America about 1870 and soon thereafter it began stimulating improvement in practice and educational programmes. In 1899, Teachers College at Columbia University offered a university-based programme to prepare teachers for schools of nursing. In 1910, the University of Minnesota established the first basic school of nursing to become part of a university system in the United States. Since that time, a series of reports and recommendations have resulted in a constant upgrading of nursing education. Significant milestones in this regard are those produced by Josephine Goldmark in 1923, Ester L. Brown in 1948, and Helen Mussallem in 1962.

During the long period of gradual improvement into the late 1940s, there was little change in the composition of the hospital staff or in the interrelationships of its members. As the person directly responsible for the care of the patient, the physician had maintained his role as the captain of the team. The nurse still functioned in a so-called "handmaiden" relationship to him and did for the patient whatever part of the therapy the doctors did not wish to undertake. One of these functions continued to be administration. Even though relationships with governments and community agencies were becoming more complex, a senior nurse, with the assistance of some clerks and aides, was expected to maintain adequate management control over the affairs of most hospitals. A few of the larger institutions were fortunate enough to obtain the services of medical or lay administrators with some formal preparation in general administration, but this was the exception rather than the rule.

The end of World War II can be marked as the point at which health care in hospitals began to move out of the fragmented cottage-industry pattern into the systems approach which attempts to make the most effective use of people and things. As is so often the case, these improved methods began first in the armed forces. Faced with extreme shortages of qualified professional personnel, and with rapidly mounting numbers of casualties, those charged with the responsibility for patient care launched into programmes for the development of a wide variety of assistants. It soon became apparent that large numbers of keen young people from many unrelated walks of life could be trained relatively quickly to become competent assistants to the members of the professional staff. These assistants carried out technical and repetitive procedures under the supervision of professionals. This enabled the doctors and nurses to devote their time to procedures requiring their level of competence and training.

The enthusiasm of ex-service personnel for such assistants or technicians was not shared by many of their civilian counterparts or by some professional associations. In the immediate post-war era, hospitals as well were slow to accept this concept. This probably resulted from the fact that, whereas in service life the roles of the doctor, the nurse, and the various assistants were clearly delineated, such was not the case in the community. Professional associations have persisted in adopting a negative attitude toward this problem. They prefer to say what a professional person is not rather than what he is. As a result, there are troublesome grey areas of responsibility between medicine and nursing, and between the professionals and their technical assistants. Each level tends to slough off procedures they no longer wish to do rather than develop positively identified fields in which they wish to work.

The result is the present situation in which we find many skilled personnel routinely carrying out activities that are far below their levels of competence. The obvious inefficiency of such a system became apparent to many thinking people during the early fifties. Fortunately, this group, which was searching for methods of improving health care, included a number of nursing educators with vision and foresight.

For over fifty years, university schools of nursing have been offering degree programmes to those who have the desire and ability to develop advanced and specialized skills. Although the organizational pattern of these schools has varied considerably in the various centres, they have all tended to develop in isolation. This has become a problem during recent years when a concerted attempt has been made to develop a team approach to patient-centred health care. Excellent programmes have been provided in a number of nursing specialties but they have tended to be heavily weighted toward the administrative and teaching specialties rather than toward clinical nursing. This has had obvious disadvantages from the point of view of those charged with the management of health-related services. On this basis, there has been obvious and unnecessary resistance to degree programmes from other sectors of the health field. It is to the eternal credit of dedicated educators like Kathleen Russell and Florence Emory of the University of Toronto School of Nursing that the degree programmes survived against such odds.

Some of these objections have been based on fact, whereas others have developed on the basis of suspicion, defensiveness, and a lack of information. The primary objection has been to the relative isolation of these schools from other university or hospital-based educational programmes in the health sciences. As often as not, this has been found to result from the attitudes of the other educational programmes rather than from a planned isolation on the part of the university school of nursing. Another objection has been the failure of many degree programmes to recognize health science education and experience at a lower level as an acceptable, and perhaps desirable, prerequisite for entrance. Such preparation has been given little recognition as a possible substitute for some of the compulsory entrance requirements. Less valid but most troublesome has been the concern of many service-oriented personnel that an effort was being made to flood the market with "chiefs" at the expense of the "Indians." These real and imaginary concerns have in the past interfered with the orderly development and expansion of higher education in nursing.

A forward step was taken in 1951 when the first associate degree programmes were started in the United States. This strengthened the belief held by many people within the nursing profession, and outside it, that the formal education system should become more involved in the preparation of health personnel. It, as well, supplemented and strengthened the stand of supporters of an expanded degree programme for professional nurses. Unfortunately, it was looked upon as a threat by many of those engaged in diploma programmes at community hospitals and it met with a lot of organized resistance. While this resistance has gradually decreased over the years, it is still evident in many areas at both the individual hospital and the health-related association levels.

The first really positive step toward the identification of the future educational and service roles of nurses in Canada was taken by Dr. Helen K. Mussallem in her thesis, "A Path to Quality," written in 1962 for her doctorate in nursing. It pointed out the necessity of avoiding the proliferation of workers in nursing with various levels of training and education. It recommended that for the future two clearly identifiable types of nurses be developed – one professional and one technical. The former should be university-educated and the latter should receive the academic portion of her programme in an educational rather than a service institution. Both should receive the clinical portions of their curricula in approved, affiliated hospitals.

These recommendations were well received by organized nursing and became the basis for the submission of the Canadian Nurses' Association to the Royal Commission on Health Services in 1964. Dr. Mussallem undertook a detailed study of Nursing in Canada for the Royal Commission. Although the report of this commission did not go so far as to rule out the need for well-trained nursing assistants, it did strongly support a marked increase in schools offering degree programmes. It also recommended that the length of diploma programmes be decreased to two years with a proportionate decrease in the service-oriented apprenticeship. This has been generally accepted as the most appropriate pattern for the future by the majority of administrators in the health field.

That is where we stand as this is written. Our projections for the future must be based on the policies and facts that are known today and the changes in systems and patterns of practice that we believe will be necessary to meet the needs of the future.

During the past ten years, administrative management has become a much stronger influence in hospitals and in the health field generally.* With government funds becoming increasingly involved in the operation of both educational and service organizations, it is obvious that as a control measure such influence will continue to increase. Hospital administration is rapidly broadening into management in the true industrial sense. In recent years, it has made increasing use of the management tools and techniques which have proven themselves in industry. It is for this reason that a more realistic and co-operative relationship between medicine, nursing, and administration is essential. If this does not develop voluntarily, it will undoubtedly be enforced legislatively at some time in the future.

A tried and true industrial management tool which has been given very little recognition in the development of educational programmes in health is marketing research. Industry has found by bitter and costly experience that it is disastrous to produce a product that is not acceptable to the public. In the past, we in the various health disciplines have adopted the "Mother knows best" attitude and have sold our products on the basis of the vague commodity known as "better patient care." There are distinct indications that a more sophisticated public and a more knowledgeable group of public servants and administrators are no longer willing to accept whatever we have to offer. It is therefore necessary that educators become completely aware of the duties and responsibilities that will be assigned to health personnel in the future, before curricula are developed for them. It also means that we can no longer afford to get locked into a rigid, unchangeable educational system that cannot react promptly to changing needs.

The systems for delivering the health services of the future will undoubtedly be centralized on a regional basis using the community

---

* This requires educational preparation that is at present not given adequate recognition in professional health sciences curricula.

hospital as a core. From the hospital the health services will extend out into the community. The community hospitals will in turn relate to teaching hospitals and other very specialized units in which the more exotic consultative and therapeutic services will be available. A team approach to comprehensive health care will be essential in such a system. The three major elements of the system – medicine, nursing, and administration – will have to be closely related at all levels. Each of these major disciplines will in turn be required to build in a much more effective interrelationship between the professional, technical, and assistant levels than they have at present. As team leader, the professional will be the thinker, planner, and organizer. The technical person will be a think-doer with a considerable scope in direct patient care and an ability to direct the activities of others. The assistants will be the doers who can be trusted to carry out a wide variety of repetitive procedures under supervision.

Such a close working relationship between various levels of personnel can be accomplished only if each group is completely aware of the areas and levels of competence of all the others. Only under such circumstances can there be a proper differentiation and delegation of responsibility for health care. Each group must have a well-defined area of knowledge and competence in which it can perform safely and efficiently. This can only be accomplished if they are brought together as students at some stage of their educational programmes, probably during part of the clinical education period. In this way, they will become aware of the special abilities of their fellow workers early in their careers and will respect these particular skills. The close co-ordination of health-related educational programmes on an interdisciplinary and intradisciplinary basis will therefore be mandatory.

Such close co-ordination can best be fostered in an organized health sciences centre programme. Such a centre need not be developed as one geographic unit so long as the related components are not too widely separated. However, on an organizational basis for educational purposes, they must function as one unit. There must be direct organizational relationship between the faculties, schools, institutes, and clinical facilities involved in the health sciences education programmes of each regional centre to ensure a co-ordinated and balanced programme. This is beginning to emerge in many areas through the grouping of health-oriented faculties and schools in a university centre under a vice-president, health sciences.

Through provincial and state departments of education and departments of health, the university-oriented programmes may in turn be co-ordinated by those provided in community colleges and institutes of technology. The melding of the various groups should occur in the affiliated teaching hospitals where the skills of the various disciplines are directed toward one primary objective – the care of the patient.

Recognition must be given to the special skills of the senior personnel involved in the service, education, and research components of such a centre. This recognition is best given by the assignment to them of the responsibilities for which they are best qualified. Good clinical, educational, and research programmes can be developed only on a solid base of excellent patient care. The administrative personnel and clinical teachers working in teaching hospitals are the experts in this field, and the responsibility for this part of the programme should be assigned to them. The well-trained administrators and teachers in the educational institutions are the experts in their special field and the educational responsibility for all programmes should be theirs. The best possible result will be achieved and the most effective use made of all facilities, if the educational responsibilities are assigned to the educational system and the provision of service and clinical experience remains with the health system.

Experience in several centres in which such a co-ordinated programme has been developed indicates that at both the professional and technological levels, it is possible to develop a basic core curriculum that is common to a number of disciplines. The sharing of this educational experience early in their careers makes each student more aware of the capabilities of others as they separate into their more specialized disciplinary fields in the academic portions of their educational programmes. A similar team approach to clinical education can and should be undertaken at the teaching hospital.

It appears likely that the responsibility for the education of personnel at a professional level in all health disciplines will be assigned to health science divisions of universities, or to special departments of community colleges closely related to, and generally supervised by, such health science divisions. Technological and technical personnel will receive their basic educational programmes either in schools of community medicine, in universities, in community colleges, or in institutes of technology. To achieve the benefits of close relationships with other technologies these schools should remain within the general education stream. Depending on specific requirements, the assistant level will be educated in centralized programmes in any one of the educational institutions mentioned above.

The various educational streams will join in the clinical atmosphere of the teaching hospital. Here each individual will be taught to work with, and to respect the special abilities of, all other members of the team in attaining the ultimate goal of all concerned – the care of the patient. Under such a system, no faculty or school can function in isolation and produce a product that is neither required nor marketable. Each student will benefit under such a programme through the concentration of educational resources and the proper orientation to his future role. Each faculty, school, and teaching hospital will enjoy the ability to concentrate all of its resources on the part of the programme which it is best qualified to handle. The economy of the nation will benefit through the avoidance of duplicating costly facilities and will, in addition, receive the advantages of better health care. Most important of all, the patient will reap the major reward of better care provided personally and efficiently through the co-ordinated efforts of a team of experts working together for a common cause.

The need for "marketing research" has been mentioned. What sort of a nurse practitioner is required for the future? It is the stated purpose of hospitals to remove as many non-nursing functions as possible from the practising clinical nurse. She will therefore be involved almost totally in direct patient care. Technology has made it impossible for any one person in the health field to be all things to all people. The days of the general practitioner in nursing are therefore numbered. As an undergraduate, the clinical nurse of the future will receive a basic two-year programme with the accent on biological and social sciences. Following this, she will be required to undertake, at the postgraduate level, an organized educational programme designed to fit her for the role she selects – bedside nursing, specialized nursing, e.g., obstetrical, psychiatric, paediatric, or intensive-care, requiring the use of special mechanical or technological equipment. Her educational programme and the management of the nursing units to which she is assigned will be directed by nursing personnel with university preparation in those specialized fields. In most specialized areas, her clinical practice will be supervised by a clinical specialist with a master's degree in her specialty. Provision will be made in the educational programmes of the future for all nurses with the ability and the desire to do so to progress from the diploma level through the various university specialties in clinical, managerial, and educational fields.

This prediction for the future may sound Utopian. It is made with due respect for the efforts of those who have worked hard in the past to develop the educational and service programmes we have today. They have striven, often against heavy odds, to develop the curricula and the service organizations which they believed would best serve the needs of patients and hospitals. The system and not the individual has been at fault. The achievement of the goal that is visualized for the future will require change on a traditional basis, and change is often painful. However, change is also inevitable if progress is to be made. Voluntary change on a co-operative basis is less traumatic than compulsory change dictated from outside the organization. The health services have not failed the citizens of our country in the past. That is the solid base that will support our hopes and aspirations for the future.

9
The education of the public health nurse

JEAN C. LEASK

The year 1920 marks the beginning of formal preparation for public health nursing in Canada. To the pioneers of the previous two decades, working as visiting nurses in the follow-up care of the tuberculosis patient, in schools, and in clinics, we owe the recognition of the potential of the nurse as a member of the public health team. The challenge and impetus of the public health movement at the close of the First World War, with its emphasis on the prevention of illness and the promotion of health, found her already working directly with families in the community and made her the logical person to undertake the role of health teaching. To fulfil this role, the need for knowledge and skills in addition to hospital preparation resulted in the establishment of a public health nursing course, one academic year in length, first at the University of Toronto and then at a number of university schools of nursing.

Two decisions made at that time by leaders in nursing had an impact on nursing education and nursing service. The first, the placement of the course in a university setting, not only established the level at which this preparation has continued to be given, but made it possible for this preparation to be enriched through the resources of other faculties within the university, particularly in the health sciences and the humanities. Certificate courses for registered nurses were the forerunners of degree programmes and have played a part in their evolution. This type of course has been the avenue through which the majority of public health nurses have entered the field of public health. The future of these programmes is a matter of considerable debate at the present time. The second decision, made on the part of the employing agencies, both public and voluntary, was to accept this educational programme set in universities, as the basic requirement for public health nursing work. Prior to this, agencies had attempted to meet the needs of staff for community work through short courses within their own organizations. This decision established the importance of the teaching function of the nurse in her work with individuals and families. The acceptance of a common preparation has contributed to the nurse's understanding of the work being carried on by her colleagues in other public health agencies and to the planning and co-ordination of public health nursing programmes. It has also been a factor in the recruitment of staff because of the ability of the nurse with this common preparation to move from one type of programme to another.

Numerically speaking, public health nurses are a relatively small segment of the total number of nurses practising in Canada, but they are the largest single group of professional workers in the public health field. Their preparation and availability for employment in the community is of vital importance to the quality of service given and to the acceptance of the responsibilities they will be asked to assume in the future.

"The purpose of public health effort," states one writer, "might be described as bringing to bear in a synthesized way, all the available scientific, educational and social skills, knowledge and discoveries so they become operative promptly as agents for the betterment of individual, family and community health."[1] The role and function of the public health nurse in the achievement of this purpose must be a constantly evolving one, subject to reappraisal. Her role changes by delegation of responsibilities in some areas, and extension of them in others. Since her working milieu is the community, adaptation to the scientific, social, economic, and cultural changes of the past fifty years have influenced the need for, and content of, her preparation. The rise in the level of general education has contributed to a public much better informed in health matters.

The changes in social attitudes toward health care have produced a demand for services to be available on a much broader base to anyone in the population, according to need rather than financial ability to secure them. This comprehensive health care is, in the opinion of one director of a public health nursing agency, more than "something of everything" in the broad spectrum of health services. It involves the putting together of the various components of health care in such a way that attention converges on the patient, his family, and the community.[2] In this context the family-centred approach of the public health nurse is reaffirmed.

The programmes carried by the first public health nurses centred for the most part around maternal and child health, school service, tuberculosis, and the care of patients at home. The health team consisted of the physician, the nurse, and, in some instances, the public health inspector. The community in which she worked, either urban or rural, usually had well-defined boundaries and a relatively simple governmental structure. Often both she and the families she served remained in this community over a period of years. The urgent need to develop the preventive aspects of health care created a division between preventive and curative services and the educational requirements for the job were clearly defined.

Today the traditional programmes have been altered, in some instances by different methods of approach, in others by a diminishing need for service as the result of advances in medical knowledge. Group teaching, not only for maternal and child health, but for the adolescent and the adult, has meant the development of new leadership skills. The public health nurse now functions in a wide variety of programmes, including mental health and the accompanying follow-up of mental illness, the care of the disabled of all ages, chronic illness, rehabilitation nursing, and the care of the rapidly increasing population in the older age group. Occupational health nursing has developed in industry, business establishments, and groups of employed workers in such settings as hospitals and government at municipal, provincial, or national levels. No longer is the line drawn between the preventive and curative aspects of care, and in modern health care there is an increasing effort being made by hospitals and public health agencies to provide continuity of care between the institution and the home, the home and the institution.

The realization that many patients with acute, chronic, or convalescent illness could be cared for at home and allow for the better utilization of hospital beds has led to the development of co-ordinated home-care programmes. In these developments, public health nurses are acting in a liaison capacity between the hospital and the community, as nurse administrators in these programmes as well as nurses giving direct care to patients. One of the most recent and interesting developments in the extension of the role of the public health nurse has been her assignment to a group of physicians in family practice, a development which will no doubt be expanded both in terms of numbers of programmes of this type and in the functions which the public health nurse will assume.

The health-care team in which the public health nurse functions has a wide variety of health workers to whom she relates either within her own organizational structure or in other allied agencies with which her programme must be co-ordinated. Today the public health nurse may work alone in a community and assume many of the functions normally carried by physicians. At the other extreme, she may be part of a highly complex urban organizational structure with all its ramifications for planning and co-ordinating health services. Increasingly, public health nursing personnel are contributing to the planning not only of their own services, but of the comprehensive health care which is emerging. Both the mobility of families and the mobility of public health nursing staff are now a fact of life in our modern society. Both have had an impact on the service given and received.

A definition of public health nursing adopted by the National League for Nursing of the United States in May 1959 and reprinted in *A Statement of Functions and Qualifications for the Practice of Public Health Nursing in Canada* is as follows: "Public health nursing is a field of specialization within both professional nursing and the broad area of organized public health practice. It utilizes the philosophy, content, and methods of public health and the knowledge and skills of professional nursing. It is responsible for the provision of nursing service on a family-centred basis for individuals and groups, at home, at work, at schools, and in public health centres. Public Health nursing interweaves its services with those of other health and allied workers, and participates in the planning and implementation of community health programs."[8]

The public health nurse of today must have a sound background of scientific knowledge; she may require the technical competence to care for patients with all types of illness and often requiring complicated treatments; in her role as a health teacher she needs the skill to impart her knowledge to a public which is now much better informed in health matters and has an increasing expectation for better health care. To assess the nursing needs of patients, observe the progress toward expected goals, and deal with problem situations, she must be capable of independent judgment. As a health counsellor and family confidante, she requires a broad knowledge of human behaviour and compassion for people. In 1970 her concern is still for people, and her programmes are directed to the individual, the family, and the community. The implications of these changes and developments in service for the preparation of the public health nurse of 1970 are apparent.

The philosophy of public health nursing as stated in *A Statement of Functions and Qualifications for the Practice of Public Health Nursing in Canada* includes the beliefs that nurses with the designated qualification of public health nurse need special preparation in order to fulfil their responsibilities, that such preparation cannot remain static if we are to adjust at the service level to meet the changing needs and demands for health care, and that there is a need for nursing personnel with different levels of preparation within the public health nursing programme. In addition to public health nursing positions at staff, supervisory, administrative, and consultant levels, the document outlines the functions of registered nurses and nursing assistants. This statement was prepared by a committee of public health nurses representing both education and service functions.

In this approach to the provision of service in the community, the various types of personnel would work as a team, led by staff public health nurses and with functions delegated to team members according to their preparation, ability, and experience. For many years the goal of all public health nursing agencies was to have all staff with public health nursing qualifications, and the standards for employment were based on this premise. This goal was achieved in some areas of Canada. In others, registered nurses were employed as temporary staff or trainees, usually with the understanding that they would pursue a course in public health nursing within a time limit. It is now realized that not only is the supply of personnel prepared for public health unable to meet all the demands of rapidly expanding community programmes, but also the skills of the public health nurse, gained through her preparation, must be used effectively. This realization will be a factor in future planning. It has been influenced by developments in nursing education.

In the fifty years, 1920 to 1970, these developments have been far-reaching. Three factors in these developments are perhaps of special significance for public health nursing. Public health nursing began as a specialty of the nursing profession, as an addition to the basic training given in a hospital school of nursing in which the focus was mainly on caring for the sick. Recognition that the individual cannot be separated from the family, friends, and the community from which he comes and to which he will return, and that the concepts of the promotion of health and the prevention of illness should precede or be integrated with the curative aspects, has gradually changed the approach to nursing education both at the diploma level and in university programmes. This change has been more rapid in the universities, but the new and re-organized programmes in diploma schools, now moving into educational settings, are incorporating these concepts into their curricula.

Realization of the need for a broad educational background to function in the role which was developing for them, has led many registered nurses to seek additional preparation at a university level and has influenced the establishment of programmes for basic nursing education within the university setting. Today, while the preparation accepted for qualification as a public health nurse continues to be in a university school, it is moving from the certificate level to that of the baccalaureate degree. We are progressing also toward the integration of preventive and curative care. The nurse now graduating with a baccalaureate degree in nursing from a basic programme and from some post-basic programmes, is being prepared to nurse either in the hospital or community setting. It is expected that in the future, preparation for public health nursing at this level will be an integral part of the nurse's education rather than a specialty.

A third factor is the movement toward the implementation of a recommendation, made by the Royal Commission on Health Services and supported by the Canadian Nurses' Association, that two categories of nurses be prepared, one at a degree level in a university programme, the other in a diploma programme, with 25 per cent of all nurses coming from the university and 75 per cent coming from diploma schools. The goal for university preparation being far short of achievement, university schools of nursing began to concentrate their efforts and resources on programmes of degree status. The implications of this for public health nursing are several.

The announcement of the discontinuance of the certificate course in public health nursing by a few university schools and its possible "phasing out" by others immediately raised the question of how standards could be maintained in the field if the main source of prepared staff was removed. It was suggested that this type of preparation be continued in another educational setting. To some of us in the service field who have urged that public health concepts be integrated into the general education of the nurse, and who had accepted the opinion of nurse educators that a certificate course based on their addition was not educationally sound, this suggestion seemed to be perpetuating a method of preparation which would not meet future staff needs. The number of degree programmes that include public health preparation is gradually increasing, but from them are to come the candidates for positions of leadership in all fields of nursing service and education. Although graduates of newer diploma programmes have potential for staff positions in community work, their preparation has not yet been considered by the public health field to be equivalent to that of the registered nurse who also had a certificate course.

It is evident that for some time to come there will not be sufficient graduates of degree programmes to fill the requirements for public health. There is also a question of whether, both from an economic and a service standpoint, all staff positions should be filled from this level. At the present time the majority of university schools offering certificate courses have met the request of the field to continue them. To resolve the situation and to plan for the future are the main tasks both of nursing service and nursing education. They must be done together.

Reference has been made to the appropriate use of the various types of nursing personnel in providing public health nursing service. This too, is an area for mutual discussion, research, and planning by education and service if we are to achieve the purpose of nursing education in relation to preparation of personnel for the job to be performed and in the numbers required. The preparation of each type to be employed will depend on the programme being carried but one would expect that the large majority would have public health nursing qualifications. The emphasis on the teaching aspects of care in the community and the impracticability from a travel standpoint of sending more than one person into a home to perform different functions, are limiting factors in the employment of registered nurses and, to an even greater extent, of nursing assistants. At the present time the nurse with public health preparation may come to the field from a certificate course, a basic, or a post-basic degree programme. She may come with no experience in service or with several years in another field of nursing. In the team approach, these variations should be considered in the assignment of levels of responsibility. Theoretically, the team leader should be a nurse with degree preparation. From a practical standpoint, we are faced with realities such as the problem of staff turnover and the need for this person to develop her own skills through experience in a first-level position before assuming further responsibility. The length of time the nurse expects to stay in the organization as well as her abilities must be considered in her selection. The substantial cost to the field of preparing a nurse for the role of team leader cannot be overlooked. An acceptance of these realities by nursing education and by the nurses themselves may lead to a better understanding of the pattern of staffing service agencies.

Nursing education for positions beyond the staff level is also in a developing stage. In this area too, preparation for the growing function of the public health nurse in planning, administration, and supervision began with a certificate course one academic year in length. To enrol in this course a nurse must have already completed a programme of preparation as a public health nurse. Referred to as advanced preparation in public health nursing and established at the request of service agencies, this programme served for many years as the main source of personnel for supervisory positions. Still available in one university school, it has assisted the service field to utilize the leadership abilities of the public health nurse who either by choice or lack of entrance requirements, is not proceeding to a baccalaureate degree.

Today the baccalaureate degree is generally accepted as preparation for supervision for nurses in the field provided that the principles are incorporated into degree programmes. Nurses with a Master's degree are still comparatively few in relation to the total work force and are, for the most part, employed in senior administrative or consultative positions. Programmes at this level are a recent development in Canada and as yet are few in number with the result that the majority of personnel with this qualification have obtained it in the United States either in university schools of nursing or in schools of public health. The cost of obtaining this preparation in another country even with bursary assistance is a deterrent to many nurses.

In the opinion of many nurse educators, preparation for supervision and administration should be at the Master's level; the present supervisor would become then a clinical specialist, highly skilled as a nurse and able to demonstrate and teach excellence in nursing care. To administrators, who even now are struggling to attain the standard of a baccalaureate degree for these positions, this goal seems unrealistic. However, as a concept it should be given thoughtful consideration today, if we are to plan for the future. In the light of changes and developments both in nursing education and service, the traditional role of the supervisor is being examined and assessed. In public health, a nursing staff which is much better prepared should be accepting more responsibility for independent action. Delegation of much of the administrative detail to clerical personnel and the use of the computer, data processing, and new methods of recording should free her to move from the office into the community as an expert advisor to staff. For the ultimate fulfilment of these goals, opportunities for the pursuit of graduate study by nurses in Canadian universities will need to increase both in numbers of programmes and areas of specialization.

In addition to the formal, academic courses of nursing education, much has been accomplished through the years by programmes of orientation and staff education given within the employing agency and through refresher courses, institutes, or seminars given under a variety of auspices including universities and professional nursing associations. This type of nursing education has been of great value in the introduction of staff to specific agency policies and procedures, in the introduction of new programmes, and in the development of new skills. Through them, nurses in the field and nurses returning to the field after several years' absence have been brought up to date in the changes in scientific knowledge which they, in turn, must incorporate into their teaching. Continuing education for the nurse, as for the members of all professions, is of increasing importance today in preparing her to meet the challenge of her changing function in the expansion of health services. In the development of programmes for nursing education, the availability of service resources is an important consideration, not only in relation to the number of students which can be accepted, but also in relation to the quality of the field experience. With the establishment of the initial course for the preparation of public health nurses, employing agencies accepted the responsibility of assisting in this preparation through the provision of field-work opportunities. For a number of years this did not present too many difficulties. The general pattern for field work was a block of several weeks in a public health nursing agency. It included observation and independent practice with supervision and evaluation by the agency staff. In this type of experience the student followed the policies and procedures of the particular agency to which she was assigned and thus she required a less detailed orientation on employment.

Many factors have contributed to the changes and modifications which have been made over the past fifty years. These have included the increasing number of students to be placed, as university certificate and degree courses developed, and the changes in philosophy and objectives of educational programmes. While a block experience is still requested and provided for some students, the length of the experience has been reduced. Concurrent field work is replacing the block pattern, particularly for preparation in basic degree programmes, and the faculty members of university schools are increasingly accepting responsibility for the supervision of the student. Since concurrent field work must be given in agencies situated in or adjacent to the city in which the university is located, the field resources are limited. As a result of these changes and modifications the purpose of field experience has been evaluated and redefined. It is now less service oriented and more directed to the application of the principles learned in academic courses through an experience of working with carefully selected individuals and families in the community. Because of difficulty in finding adequate resources for field experience for all students, the possibility of its discontinuance has been discussed and this step has been taken in one certificate programme. If adequate field resources are not available, there would seem to be no alternative but to further reduce or modify this experience.

Public health nursing agencies have always given priority to students in public health nursing programmes, but the demands for student observation from diploma schools of nursing are constantly increasing. Having accepted that their courses should incorporate the concepts of public health, their desire for the student to observe in the community is a natural result. Here again the numbers who can be given this opportunity are limited. Often the largest diploma schools of nursing are located in the same centres as university schools and the same field resources must be used. Methods of providing field experience will continue to be a problem area. In my opinion the association of a student with a field agency is a valuable one to retain and it would be hoped that we who are in the field can continue to work with nursing education at all levels in providing an experience which will meet their objectives and at the same time be within the limits of our resources.

At this point in our development as a profession we are looking toward a future in which the expansion of health services will make greater demands on our resources, a future in which the changes of the past fifty years may seem small by comparison. One of the main considerations of the planners for health services today is to decide how and by whom these services will be delivered to the people who require them. It is predicted that many more people will receive these services at home and that many more nurses will be working in the community setting. The people who require these services live not only in cities but in rural areas and isolated communities. Unless nurses as individuals and the profession as a whole are willing to work toward the provision of our service to all these areas in the amount that is required, we will be failing in our responsibility and relinquishing our function to other workers.

The nurse who will meet the challenge of the future is better pre-pared for her role. Taught to inquire rather than accept, from an approach based on learning the principles of care rather than just procedures, she should be ready to adapt to the changes ahead. The role and function of the public health nurse of 1970 have been greatly expanded as compared with those of the nurse of 1920. There is no doubt that this role will continue to be extended if we are willing to reach out to new fields of service instead of simply allowing our functions to evolve with the changes in other profes-sions, particularly medicine. The nursing profession should be an active participant in planning for the assumption of additional re-sponsibilities and for the inherent preparation required.

Today a great deal of emphasis is given to the team approach. In the nursing care of patients in the community the basic team is the nurse, the patient, and the family. The nurse who goes to the home is responsible for the total nursing care required at that time, which may include both a complicated treatment and a simple procedure. In this ability to complete the total care that is necessary the nurse finds great satisfaction. It may be a contributing factor in the de-sire of the majority of nurses in the community to remain in positions involving direct patient care.

We must constantly remember that nursing education is not an end in itself but a beginning for service; that service agencies do not exist primarily for the employment of individuals but for the provision of health care. I believe the public will support the aims of nursing education and service if our goals are directed to the improvement of the nursing care we give and if we do, in fact, produce a type of nursing care which will meet their expectations. Nursing education and nursing service must work as a team to achieve these goals. For the goal of integration of the nurse's function with those of other professions in future health programmes, the team in both education and service will need to be representative of the professions that will be working together. Perhaps one of the problems of co-ordinating the services given by various health workers has been the almost complete separation in the preparation of the various disciplines. In speaking of public health, it is the opinion of Dr. John Hastings that if we are to develop this field of work to meet the modern and future problems of health care we must begin to think of ourselves, not primarily as physicians, nurses, dentists, etc., but as public health professionals who happen to have a medical, nursing, dental, or other basic preparation.[4] The integration of some courses for workers in the health field at the educational level would, I believe, lead to a better co-ordination of service programmes in the community.

It has been said that the way to honour pioneers is to pioneer. The nursing pioneers of 1920 envisaged the place of the nurse in the development of public health at that time. The graduates of today will be the pioneers of tomorrow. They must also look to the future but it will be in relation to the place of the nurse in comprehensive health care in a highly complex society.

NOTES

1 Ruth B. Freemen, "Team Work in Public Health," *Canadian Journal of Public Health* (September 1964): 381.
2 Eva M. Reise, "Public Health Nursing and Comprehensive Health Care," *Nursing Outlook* (January 1968): 48.
3 Canadian Public Health Association, *A Statement of Functions and Qualifications for the Practice of Public Health Nursing in Canada,* October 1966, p. 2.
4 John E. Hastings, "Some Plain Thoughts on the State of Public Health," *Canadian Journal of Public Health* (March 1969).

10
A general practitioner considers nursing education

MORLEY A. R. YOUNG

George Santayana has said, "He who is disposed to ignore history, must be prepared to relive it." This book covers a period of fifty years in the field of nursing, much of it with an historical implication. In many areas of human endeavour fifty years would be but as a few minutes in one's life time. In nursing as we know it today, fifty years is almost half the period of its existence. It is long enough to warrant a look back as well as ahead. We give heed to Santayana's observation.

The status of the general practitioner would appear to be of less importance today than it was in the years gone by. Fifty years ago the general practitioner was "the doctor." He did his best to look after the ills of humanity. He sought advice and assistance, at times, from a confrère who had a special interest in some particular field. Then specialism began to develop and in many areas of medical practice the doctor limited his efforts to a restricted field. He concentrated his study and training accordingly. More and more specialists appeared in the field of medical practice and the general practitioner for a time seemed to be of less importance. Today it is again abundantly clear that the general practitioner is needed in the practice of medicine. It has been said on many occasions that a good general practitioner could adequately look after more than three-quarters of the current ills of our patients, leaving the balance to the specialists. There is also the continuing need for the care of the patient as a total human being.

The nursing profession is travelling a trail similar to that taken by the medical profession from general practitioners to specialists to a renewed demand for general practitioners. We used to have bedside nurses who gave total patient care, to the best of their ability, to all patients. The need for some nurses with special education and training became obvious and this was met and rightly so. Now we have the specialists. Could history have something to say to us here?

In 1920, when the Toronto School began its work, there was in the field of illness a trinity whose services were obviously needed and whose activities covered quite a wide area in the health field. This trinity was made up of the patient, the doctor, and the nurse. This unit, although somewhat hidden by para-personnel, is still with us and must be, many of us believe, for some years to come. It was in this setting that the image of The Nurse was born. After fifty years this image of the nurse may have faded somewhat, but it is still quite easily seen. In another fifty years something different may be in its place.

Another facet of this image of the nurse is the private-duty nurse. Prior to World War II this type of nursing was much more common than in the years that followed. During the first decade after the war many members of any class graduating from a school of nursing planned to do private-duty nursing. Today almost every member of such a class is looking for an institutional position. In the sphere of private-duty nursing, either in the home or in the hospital, there was an excellent opportunity for a patient-doctor-nurse relationship. The general practitioner, and others, in thinking about nursing education may be influenced in his thinking by an image of the nurse acquired years ago, and which has not yet faded from memory.

The field of general education in Canada today seems to be plagued with controversy. Discussions centre around both method and content. The purpose of many forms of education is viewed and reviewed. There is an effort to produce an educated individual who will be able to cope with the demands of this mechanistic and frustrated age. Nursing education is no exception, and much change has taken place over the fifty years. In 1920 the major portion of the nurse's education was given by the apprenticeship method. Today more and more of it is developed in the collegiate atmosphere. The slower method of learning by doing has given way to the do-by-learning process. As in many other areas of life, needs and demands have brought about characteristics of mass production.

One could discuss at length the advantages and disadvantages of one method as compared with the other. Personally I feel that, while much has been gained, more than a little has been lost. An important item of loss is the patient-doctor-nurse relationship.

Many changes and developments have taken place in the sphere of nursing education. Most of the schools of nursing have been hospital-based schools granting diplomas after a successful three-year course. Education beyond this level was university-based. Many nurses have graduated from our hospital schools and are active in the broad health field. Many of the leaders in nursing have come to us from the hospital-based school. We have had a good system, but hoping for a better one has brought about change.

Two areas showing very definite change are noted in a comparison of nursing education of the 1920s with that of the 1960s. In the first place there is a marked increase in the number of hours that the student spends in the classroom in collegiate surroundings. In the second place there is an almost corresponding decrease in the hours that the student spends on the wards and associated with the patients. A review was taken at three different periods over the last fifty years, considering the curriculum and programme of education in one of the smaller schools. The extent of change will become very clear. The data were from three three-year periods which ended in the years 1921, 1945, and 1968, respectively. The 1921 record summarizes the practical work as follows: men's surgical, 279 days, women's surgical and obstetrical, 270 days, children and medical, 288 days, operating and delivery room, 110 days, night supervisor, 103 days, vacations and sick leave, 46 days (vacation 2 weeks each year). Being a scrub nurse for 71 operations was required. Then the theoretical work and examinations were recorded: the doctors lectured in surgery, gynaecology, orthopaedics, bandaging and operating-room techniques, obstetrics, paediatrics, venereal diseases, anatomy and physiology, materia medica, urinalysis, and bacteriology; the superintendent of nursing and her assistant took care of practical nursing, ethics and the history of nursing, obstetrics, dietetics, and materia medica. Total time for lectures was 104 hours. It is noted that bacteriology was allocated 3 hours.

Drawing a 1945 record from the files there is a noticeable change. A record of the number of hours of instruction comes first, distributed as follows: preliminary term, 188 hours, junior term, 169 hours, intermediate term, 128 hours, and the senior term, 85 hours, making a total of 570 hours of classroom work. A summary of the practical work makes a total of 1,096 days, which is the same as in 1921. It is obvious that if the student is in class she is not on the ward. The number of subjects taught has doubled and the major part of the instruction is carried out by specially trained nursing personnel. In this school the doctors still lecture but the relative number of hours is much reduced.

The record reviewed for 1968 shows a further change in the direction already noticed. The hours given to lectures, and laboratory and clinical teaching total 1,467. These hours are distributed among 27 subjects or courses. The summary of the clinical experience days totalled for the three years gives a figure of 776 days. These figures are from the three-year diploma course. There may seem to be some discrepancy in the number of days recorded but the last total of days does not include affiliations and some deductions for a block programme. I think it is obvious from the examples that the trend in nursing education has been away from the wards and into the classroom.

It is on the floors of the hospitals whose capacity is one hundred beds or less that the general practitioner is found and the doctor-nurse relationship established. Here the doctor may estimate or determine the trends in nursing education. This he does from his contact with the finished product, so to speak, although there are still a number of these hospitals that operate schools of nursing. In these schools doctors still do some of the teaching and lecturing. But whether or not the doctor takes part in the teaching programme, the fact that he is associated with a hospital having a school of nursing gives the general practitioner some direct knowledge of the curriculum and he is aware of the trends in teaching the nursing student.

I interviewed personally twenty-five active general practitioners from both urban and rural settings, discussing with them nursing education. Their comments were based either on direct knowledge of curriculum content and teaching practices, or on inferences drawn from their experience in working with nurses who have graduated in recent times from our schools. In noting the qualities of today's nurse it was inevitable that some comparisons would be made with nurses of the past. The image of the nurse held by a good number of doctors, however, is not necessarily compatible with the trends in nursing education today. It is disturbing to find that only 20 per cent of the doctors interviewed complimented the recent graduate on being a good nurse and were happy with her attitudes, her work, and her assistance. The remainder were more or less critical of the work the nurse was doing. They felt that there were deficiencies in her education and training. To them the nurse was a member of the health team of which the doctor was the leader and where the patient-doctor-nurse relationship was an important feature.

Those practitioners who had some knowledge of nursing education and its trends expressed some concern that the leaders in the nursing field did not appear to be basically in agreement as to where they were going or what they wished to accomplish in the field of nursing education. There was a bit of worry that there seemed to be evidence that nurses were no longer educated primarily to look after sick people. Teachers and leaders seemed to be more concerned with professional status. Patient care would thus become a means to an end rather than an end in itself. The loss of that quality produced by the patient-nurse relationship was regretted. That attribute cannot be acquired in the classroom. It was pointed out on more than one occasion that in the medical schools today the students were being introduced to the hospital ward and to the patient's bedside earlier than ever before in the history of medicine. In a sense it is there that they will remain until the time of graduation. The trend in nursing education would appear to be in the opposite direction.

At the risk of being tedious it will be well to note some of the major criticisms made by the general practitioners and make some comments in connection with most of them. There is a very definite feeling that a number of the courses offered to the student nurse are too detailed and too long. Anatomy, microbiology, psychiatry, and pharmacology were mentioned as areas where too much was given and too much expected. Particularly in psychiatry and pharmacology it was pointed out that what is accepted today may be obsolete in a year or so and is really of questionable value to the nursing student. The opinion was expressed that many of the texts were very technical and seemed to be written as a scientific treatise rather than a book from which to learn. Some were said to be as technical, if not more so, as those used in the medical schools.

Is there a basis for this opinion concerning the four subjects mentioned? Reference to the hours of instruction as listed earlier in this paper reveals the following figures for the years 1921, 1945, and 1968: in anatomy and physiology, 40, 70, and 140 hours were spent, respectively; in psychiatry, 0, 25, and 100 hours; in microbiology, 3,

19, and 43 hours; and in pharmacology, 12, 30, and 65 hours. The critical observation was that some of the courses are too detailed and too long.

A consensus of opinion existed to the effect that the younger nurse of today did not or would not accept responsibility with respect to the patient. This was given to or taken by the head nurses and administrators often by remote control so it seemed. This quality of assuming responsibility was a characteristic of our nurses until recent times. It is gradually fading from those who are now on our wards. In the same vein it was reported that many of our nurses never get to know the patient as a person. Often he is just a case or a room number. Some of the doctors remarked that they felt that many nurses were afraid to accept responsibility. The legal aspect of this situation was brought forward as a possible explanation of, or basis for, this fear.

The fear of, or failure to assume, responsibilty was most noticeable in the field of obstetrics and also where the postoperative patient was concerned. To the general practitioner in the smaller hospital this lack was a real handicap. Why has this situation developed? Consideration was given to the current educational process to determine, if possible, a cause for this lack of maturity in many of the nurses. It was pointed out that, while students, these young women were given little if any real responsibility. The doctors felt that there were too many supervisors and head nurses under whose watchful eyes the student had to work. It was felt that in the last two or three months of the course the student should have to assume definite responsibility. Only by having responsibility placed upon her would the young nurse develop confidence in herself and be able to take her place on the health team. Over the fifty years of our survey the number of classroom hours has increased 14 fold when one notes the figures for 1921 and 1968. The classroom is an excellent place to acquire knowledge but it is practical experience that builds confidence and helps to develop the ability to assume responsibility.

Associated with this thinking was a comment to the effect that the smaller school of nursing was to be complimented on the quality of nurse produced. It was stated that, because on the average they were good nurses, the demand both at home and in the United States for nurses from these schools was very pronounced. They were said to handle the patient with more assurance, were more at home in the case room, and seemed to know what to do for the patient who had returned to the ward from the recovery room. It was felt that the student from the larger school had too much supervision. This supervision lacked the personal touch, which was more apt to be present in the smaller school. This personal attention came from both the doctors and the nurses with whom the student was associated. It was granted that in these days of mass production it was a problem to know how to retain these desired qualities.

Bedside nursing was a term that came up frequently. It appears that not many nurses are interested in doing this type of work in our modern hospitals. The young woman wants to be a ward supervisor or an administrator of some type. This might be a reflection of the educational process. Perhaps the field of bedside nursing has not been stressed enough to the student during her course. Perhaps the amount of paper work or administrative detail sidetracked her. One irritated doctor referred to nurses doing charting at their desks as "pencil pushers." He wanted to know the use of tons of nurses' notes. "What a waste of effort and time" was his final comment.

There is more than a grain of truth in these various statements. The fault that develops because of this situation is that the nurse is not with the patient. It is recognized that the nurse-patient relationship is more difficult to establish in the five-day week with the ambulatory patient, but it is still part of the "nurse image." It is an important area in the field of hospital care and its retention is much to be desired.

In further discussion of the various aspects of bedside nursing it was felt that too much of this is left to the certified nursing assistant. It was thought that the nine-month course of training given these aides was not enough to prepare them for the responsibility that they often have thrust upon them. What is the answer? Either the certified nursing assistant course has to be lengthened or our schools of nursing will have to produce two categories of graduate nurses, the administrator supervisor, educated to manage the hospital ward, and the nurse prepared to do bedside care, who would be the nurse so far as the patient's wants and needs are concerned.

In this context the two-year college-based course, in its various forms, came up for a brief discussion. Accurate knowledge as to content of the various curricula was wanting. There was a very definite feeling that a nurse could not be produced in two years and that the student from such a school would require quite a number of months of supervised internship. The final product "might" be satisfactory. Most of the doctors interviewed were definitely in favour of continuing the hospital diploma nursing courses. One might note in passing that this is the type of school the doctors are familiar with and it is from here that they get their nurses.

A number of doctors contacted were from the British Isles and their expectations were at times different from ours. They had the feeling that team nursing was a term used rather than a fact expressed. This is an interesting observation to be made in Canada where we feel a good deal of progress has been made in this area. The rather frequent reference to the failure to assume responsibility or show initiative came up again. Would the nurse with these two qualities make a good team member?

Whatever it is in nursing education that results in the student developing a good patient-nurse relationship appears to be considered of less importance in nursing schools today. This is the conclusion one arrives at after talking to a good number of general practitioners. The evidence given to support this feeling is that there does not appear to be any depth or meaning in many of the functions performed by the nurse for her patient. She does not report signs or symptoms accurately. She is not interested enough in the patient, as a person, to observe him carefully. Too much reliance is put on laboratory reports and mechanical aides and not enough on judgment, human interest, and common sense. This discussion is not entirely new. However it was admitted by these men and women that the qualities they were looking for came with experience but that even so it was their opinion that many of our nurses of today do not get the proper orientation at the bedside of the patient.

Among medical men one rather frequently hears the opinion expressed that all doctors should have experience in general practice before they begin taking a training in any specialty. I gather that there is a similar feeling with respect to nurses. Those in teaching positions seemed to be the ones thought of in this connection. More than once it was suggested to me that too many of the teachers and instructors in our schools of nursing were in those positions because basically they did not like to do nursing. They were interested in teaching rather than in nursing and as a result their students got a nursing education with too much of an academic tinge. To a less extent supervisors and head nurses were also categorized in this manner. All these leaders should demonstrate their ability to "nurse" before they take any advanced education. Again, the regret was expressed that the nurse is getting too far away from the patient. From the apprenticeship method to the computer-assisted classroom is quite a step. It takes time to accommodate to the new situation. Attention was again called to the trend in medical education toward returning to the bedside. "What about nurses?" the general practitioner asks.

One could not help but note the frequency with which the general practitioner compared the nurse of former years with those of today. The comparison was not entirely favourable to our younger nurses. It may have been that the doctor felt he knew more about the education and abilities of former graduates and stressed what he knew. The statement was made that if one wants to get a good supervisor or head nurse one should not employ a recent graduate. Academic qualifications did not take first place with the speaker. His belief was that the woman who had graduated some time ago and had probably raised a family and now felt free from home duties was the one to look for. It would be necessary for her to take a refresher course (and the higher its quality the better), but having completed this she would be someone really worthwhile. She was mature, had an interest in human beings, assumed responsibility well, and would probably remain with you for some years to come. This was in contrast to the rapid change-over of staff at the present time in all hospitals. The doctor expressing these views felt that the nurses of some years ago had had a better nursing education than the young women of today.

The various comments we have taken note of stem from discussions with general practitioners. They concern the status of nursing education and they leave no doubt in the minds of these men and women that there is room for improvement. This of course must be true if we are to progress. When a doctor is asked to discuss nursing education of today he first has to establish a norm in his thinking. In such a situation it is normal in most of us to turn to the past and base our opinions on our experience, and on these we base our assessment of the present. Trying to take a careful look at the future is not an activity in which many of us are seriously engaged. So our general practitioner friends look back, remembering as a rule only the best, and by comparison the present does not look as good as it might, otherwise.

Most of the doctors still think of the nurse as a reliable assistant. She is one in whom he would like to have confidence and one who

will look after his patient when he is not there. So long as we practise curative medicine the doctor will feel the need for some such
person, because this type of work will be necessary. Nurses may
resent to a degree this "doctor's helper" title but there is such a
need and someone must fill it. Rightly or wrongly the nursing assistant is having more and more of this responsibility thrust upon her.
Nurses are well educated but one wonders if this role is stressed too
much during their course. There is the feeling that too much of an
independent course is encouraged. Patient care suffers and the
patient-doctor-nurse concept becomes rather meaningless.

At this stage in our discussion it would seem that we should ask,
"What is the considered opinion of general practitioners with respect
to nursing education?" The answer would seem to be somewhat as
follows. One-fifth of our general practitioners feel that the preparation given and the education provided must be adequate since the
product is a good nurse who is giving a fine account of herself. She
is giving the patients good care and the doctor-nurse relationship is
satisfactory. However, the majority of medical men feel otherwise.

The opinions expressed by those doctors who were not happy with
the graduates of our schools of nursing varied from the pointing out
of some weaknesses to being quite critical. Many of the opinions expressed were repeated in one interview after the other. In attempting
to pinpoint weaknesses it would seem that immaturity and a failure
to accept responsibility loomed rather prominently in their thinking.
Lack of concern for patients as human beings and a tendency to
show a spirit of selfishness were other points of criticism. These traits
resulted in below-standard patient care on the one hand and too
much concern over hours of duty and days off on the other. It is
difficult to blame these shortcomings on the educational system
under consideration. These students are the material with which the
educational system has to work. These young women are the products of our modern society and have been partially moulded before
they ever came to our schools of nursing.

In the more definite realm of the educational process itself there
was the feeling that too much effort was spent in producing a highly
educated and scientifically orientated person. The need was for more
people with human interest attributes and whose field of activity
centred around a sick person. The definite need in the nursing world
for administrators was recognized, but a familiar saying used on
more than one occasion was "There are too many chiefs and not

enough braves." It was evident that there is among our general practitioners a very strong feeling that nursing education is carried on these days too far away from the patient. Nurses cannot be developed in the classroom any more than doctors can be. The basic ingredient in a good nurse is bedside experience. One doctor expressed it this way, "The aim of nursing education should be to produce a good nurse, not necessarily a well-educated young woman."

It would be well at this point to call attention to the fact that the term "bedside nursing" has a much different connotation now than it had twenty years ago. Chemotherapy, antibiotics, and early ambulation all combine to shorten the period the average patient spends in bed. Instead of bedside nursing the nursing care that is often required might better be described as ward nursing. The fundamental need that the various doctors are indicating is that of a sound nurse-patient relationship whether it be acquired at the bedside, in the ward, or in the dayroom.

Now that the general practitioner has considered nursing education, probably somewhat superficially, has he any comments or predictions as to what the future might hold? The belief was expressed that, if present trends in nursing education continue, all bedside nursing will have to be done by certified nursing assistants. It would then be necessary to give them a better education. Their course would probably become a two-year term of educational and practical experience. The alternative to this is to produce two categories of registered nurses. One type would do the ward nursing and the other would be directed toward supervision and administration. The teaching could be the same throughout the greater part of such an undertaking. Bedside experience would be stressed as part of the educational experience. The doctor in general practice is not an educational expert. He is usually quite a practical man and his solution to many of his problems is to listen to the voice of experience. He applies the same treatment when questioned about nursing education.

I have been closely associated with nursing education all my professional life. I have seen much change, most of it for the better. The great change in the educational approach has been from that of the apprenticeship method to that of the collegiate atmosphere. I fear that the pendulum has been allowed to swing too far. In the realm of nursing education we must continue to progress by retaining from the past that which has been proven to be good, and by carefully testing that which is new in the school of experience. Throughout all this, patient or health care is our *raison d'être*. Along with many of my medical colleagues and not a few of our nurses I would hope that the hospital-based school of nursing would remain with us for many years to come.

11
The humanities in the nursing curriculum

RONALD R. PRIEST

For what are we educating the nurse? For her profession? For her future role in society as it extends beyond that profession? Or are we educating her as a human being living in a world of living people? Questions like these have confronted educational philosophers since Plato, and they confront us today when we attempt to consider the nature and role of education in the life of the nurse. Before issues can be intelligently scrutinized, however, terms must be defined, and in our context we are in the greatest danger of equivocating on that word education.

For purposes of simplification – and I admit to the problems of simplification – there are two kinds of education: there is that kind that sets out to train, to pass on a skill, or specifically qualify one for a job; and there is that kind that has as its objective the development of the whole man – intellectually, morally, and spiritually. The first kind is really vocational training, and, although at the university level in law, medicine, and engineering it is euphemistically referred to as professional training, the difference is only in degree, not in type. The second kind is education in the purer sense. It is not, I hasten to add, education for education's sake, but education for man's sake; it is not education for the good of society, either, or the good of mankind or whatever other shoddy collectives come to mind. Only in so far as society is the aggregate of men does it involve itself in building a better society through those men.

These two kinds of educational purposes, while replete with contradictions and philosophical implications in themselves, are rendered all the more obscure by their having been combined in most of our Canadian educational schemes. The marriage has proved to be an unfortunate one for instead of each partner complementing the other, the more pragmatic partner has come to dominate and use – in the worst sense of the word – the other. The results are widespread. Thousands of young men and women are entering our universities, our community colleges, and our schools of nursing to be trained for a job. If they undertake liberal or humanistic studies – and some do not – the bias and the orientation of those studies is usually designed to develop those intellectual, moral, and spiritual qualities that will reinforce job skills. Undoubtedly, the process serves the needs of industry and the practical requirements of society very well – it is efficient and it is economical. But it does not intrinsically encourage excellence, or self-knowledge, or increased awareness in the person. It makes no overt attempt to emancipate our youth from the darkness and ignorance of the human condition; it makes no attempt to broaden the narrow mind and enlarge the withered heart. It does, however, unconsciously but perniciously, subjugate them to the emptiness of twentieth-century materialism we call living.

I am not suggesting that our educational institutions have not lived up to their responsibilities as professional schools. There is a host of men and women in our society today who are performing their tasks with great skill and responsibility. But many of them are cultural and spiritual eunuchs who exude neither warmth nor sensitivity. They see their role as filling the job and because they are unable to achieve spiritual fulfilment they often compensate by becoming materialistic, status-conscious, narcissistic, and, thereby, appropriately busy. They cease, as almost all society has ceased, to be reflective and introspective and are caught in the maelstrom of secular passion we call twentieth century civilization. Our stress on technological innovation gives assurance of excellence in our professional programmes; our lack of stress on humanistic concerns denies attainment of intellectual and spiritual quality in these same individuals. We have created the modern Doctor Faustus.

Nine hundred years ago humanities students were exposed to what was known as the Latin Trivium consisting of logic, grammar, and rhetoric. These three elements frequently referred to as the language arts were not taught as subjects themselves but as integral to the approach to any material whether in philosophy, history, or theology. In this situation the student exercised his skill in logic as he acquired it, in sorting out the arguments of the masters. Similarly he learned his grammar, not by rote, but by evaluating structure, word order, and syntax in the context. Finally, as he examined the author's purposes and evaluated the methods whereby the author achieved those purposes, he became involved with rhetoric. In this manner he became steeped in every facet of the presentation of the material and hence of the material itself. The architects of these educational schemes were wise in laying stress on language study; they recognized that the avenue of all education is language. It is to our discredit that we do not structure our educational schemes around language study, because words, whether spoken or written, whether on film, live, or printed in a book, are the basic constructs by which we communicate. And to survive – physically and spiritually – we must not just communicate our science; we must also communicate our ideals and our culture.

Of course, a cure only begins in diagnosis and the cure for our educational ill can only come about if we are able to develop a new breed of teachers. We certainly do not need the specialist, zealous for his discipline and knowledgeable of its prerogatives. His exercising militates against what we are trying to do by fragmenting knowledge, by teaching the discipline for the discipline's sake as though each of his students was to become what he is in miniature. Knowledge in the real world is not fragmented and compartmentalized but linear and integrated and to convey this unity we need teachers dedicated to excellence and the pursuit of truth while eclectic in their approach. The fulfilment of that need is closer to realization if we invoke the language arts with a stress on rhetoric.

In spite of the many pejorative connotations of the word rhetoric, some of which have been acquired quite deservedly, it remains that there is much good to be derived from a revival of rhetoric, especially if the terms of reference are broadened for the modern setting and if it is examined as both an instructional and analytical tool.

In modern terms, rhetoric is the art and science of communication, and, whenever men communicate, rhetoric is involved. Because some men have studied rhetorical modes or have become steeped in them, often under other names, they are able to communicate effectively; nevertheless, all communication is rhetorical; only the quality and the degree of effectiveness vary. But someone will say, "Is not 'language' or 'communications' close to the discipline of 'English' as it is offered in our educational systems?" Undoubtedly yes, but insofar as rhetoric involves a reorganization of material and a reorientation of approach it is superior to traditional English literature and composition programmes because it retains and amplifies the cultural and humanistic concerns while expanding the language concerns. In the English speaking world we have forgotten that there was a time when there was no English literature. We would do well to reflect on that fact. For, as our literature has grown first in poetry, then drama, and, since the seventeenth century, the novel, so has the immensity of the problem in coping with it grown. Our universities have been churning out graduates in English literature who, although familiar with the technical aspects of the literature, are very often unaware of how to approach the elucidation of its values, let alone evaluate the language in which these values are cloaked.

A rhetorical approach, on the other hand, analyses the rules and strategies used by great authors as tactics in communication, and to engage in such analysis is to come closer to a full appreciation of the author's ideals and experiences. The benefits are two-fold: an increased awareness of how language can be used in shaping communication for one's ends, and the transmission of culture. A still greater advantage of rhetorical analysis is the scope of material that can be analysed. Because all communication involves rhetoric, our selection of literature need not be restricted to short stories, novels, or the essays of traditional programmes; we are free to select any literature, whether it be in political science, philosophy, history and the social sciences, or even the pure sciences. There appear to be but three limiting factors in the selection: the familiarity of the instructor with the relationship of the elements of classical rhetoric so as to relate them to the modern student; a good knowledge of the field discipline involved; and that the works exemplify the cultural and humanistic traditions we judge as essential to intellectual growth.

The critic can argue against this position from two perspectives, and, oddly enough, if one is valid the other is invalid. My point is that both are inadequate. Simply stated, the perspective is either that such an approach is in danger of diluting the real value of traditional English studies, because of the *pot pourri* of material; or, that many philosophical, sociological, and political questions are already posed in works by modern writers like Camus, Salinger, and Steinbeck, to say nothing of Shakespeare, Mill, or Shaw. The first perspective has to be unacceptable if only because it implies that truth, beauty, and goodness are restricted to the literature of a period, to a genre, or even to an author. Furthermore, since the second perspective is valid, the first is further negated. My criticism of the second is that too few teachers pursue those philosophical, socio-logical, and political questions, because they have no mode for handling them. The demands of a scholastic and academic approach by any university English department too often limits the scope of that department's programme to the environment of the text. As a result, the young adolescent, whether he or she be a student nurse or a student doctor, or a student engineer is faced with puristic ques-tions like, "Discuss the mythical imagery in *A Portrait of the Artist as a Young Man.*" "What do you know about Christopher Marlowe? Mention some of the main works and mention why he is important in English literature." "How is *Tess of the D'Urbervilles* a good example of the theme-ridden novel?" and so on *ad nauseum*. These questions are not absolutely irrelevant. Undoubtedly they, and others like them, are as germaine to the scholastic discipline of the student of English literature as the memorization of the periodic table is to the student of chemistry. But we are not teaching spe-cialists in English literature, nor is the prospective nurse a student of English literature. She is, as all educated people should be, a student of life, and what she needs is not further fragmentation of knowledge but a multidisciplinary and eclectic understanding of knowledge that will render her thinking more linear and her life more livable. A rhetorical approach can do both.

Another bonus of the utilization of rhetorical analysis is that it makes the student of language wiser about the ways of other men. It does not take much insight for one to perceive that much of life is lived amidst tensions arising from contradictions: the need for har-mony in human relationships but the potential discord built into the contrasting nature of each human personality; the obvious need for charity and sensitivity but the mass dissemination of the violent and gross in our culture; the enormous potential for the development of man's intellectual capacities through the greatly shortened work week but his enslavement to the crass commercialism and the sub-human appetites aroused by wicked men greedy for economic gain. As people professing humanistic concerns we render a great dis-service to humanity by not equipping our young men and women to detect and cope with pernicious and immoral argument. We are here, not as pedagogues ritualizing a technical language for the sake of the devoted few, but as men and women who, having learned much about life in living it, desire to teach young men and women to think and to speak, and, where necessary, to write, intelligently, morally, and forcefully about affairs affecting humanity.

One of the frightening prospects that Huxley points out in his *Brave New World* is that all that is good and human and true – which in large measure has provided the environment that generated the nature and success of our enterprise – is in danger of being swallowed up in the "great capitalist maw." As a consumer of goods under the western capitalistic market economy, man has himself become a commodity to be manipulated and consumed by our enormously powerful economic system. In our market system he has become the object of that system and is literally expected to find his salvation in the wares of the world. But man is not just the end of some system (if only because some men cannot partake of it) – man cannot live by bread alone. Within every man is the vestige – or, if you prefer, the rudiment – of the divine potential. Perhaps in the nurse it is just a little more in evidence because of the humanitarian nature of her calling. But if the educational structure does not encourage and facilitate increased awareness and realization of that fact; if the curriculum does not allow for the development and the expression of the creative imagination so that the individual can transcend himself and his environment, then we are indeed shortchanging the individual. In such a strategic function as nursing, where the nurse has yet much to fight for in terms of human dignity and already gives more than most in service to society, only the most excellent means of mental development should be offered to her. A revival of humanistic studies with a strong rhetorical emphasis offers the most valid material for such a programme.*

* For further information on the nature of the rhetorical approach to literature, the reader is advised to consult the forthcoming OISE Report of the English Study Committee on Rhetoric, due in 1970.

PART THREE   THE NEXT FIFTY YEARS

12
2020: Health services fifty years hence

JOHN D. HAMILTON

The best-trained scientist does not often give way to flights of imagination about the future, because such self-indulgence is a threat to
the disciplined logic of scientific thought. It leads in other words
to sloppy thinking, like cocktails before lunch. But given the opportunity and justification, then the brake of conscience lets go all too
quickly and the well-grounded scientist takes off into a brave new
world undreamed of by Aldous Huxley or H. G. Wells. This
Utopia must be based on the assumption, first, that human nature
can change and, second, that this will have been accomplished before the perfect world is achieved. Without these two premises the
possibility hangs over us that science unlimited may eliminate man
because of his atavistic nature.

My initial elation stimulated by the opportunity to write about
health services fifty years hence quickly died, for the change in
man's character in the past fifty years does not presage any major
changes in the next half century. One may predict that fifty years
hence civilized man will cling as tenaciously to a mode of life and
pattern of health service that he knows as he does today. In other
words, the evolution of health services during the past fifty years,
and their present structure, should give a reasonable basis for pro-
jecting modifications both desirable and possible during the next few
decades. It is safe to predict evolution of such services proceeding
faster than before in Canada, but not necessarily in other parts of
the world. I should state at this point that my remarks about the
future of health services relate only to Canada where today there
are wide differences in the kind of service available from one part
of the country to the other, but where the introduction of medicare

promises in time the development of a service more uniform in both kind and quality.

To weave a pattern for the future out of the threads of the past is logical, if the threads can be identified. In the case of health services, they must be traced from every aspect of our environment, social structure, and scientific development. Science alone is perhaps the most predictable contributor to health, so that a beginning can be made through examining what science has achieved in the prevention and treatment of disease during the past fifty years, and what it promises for the next half century.

As a starting point in the past I have chosen 1920, or, more correctly, the period following the First World War, because this was an era of consolidation and application of new knowledge in health services. It all began much earlier, in Paris, during the last two decades of the nineteenth century with the discovery by Pasteur that micro-organisms cause disease. From then up to the Second World War all the excitement in medical science was in France. In North America before 1900, only a few centres, McGill in Montreal and Johns Hopkins in Baltimore most notably, kept abreast of what was happening in Europe. Elsewhere in the United States, and to a less extent in Canada, medical education had fallen into the hands of the practising profession, with disastrous results. The physicians kept the scientific basis firmly tied to anatomy alone. By 1900, however, the University of Toronto had regained possession of medical education, planned a new curriculum and a new building and then embarked on a rising tide of development that lasted into the 1930s. By 1920, the Rockefeller Foundation had launched its programme for the advancement of public health by separating from the medical schools the education of those responsible for protection of the community from the ravages of infectious disease, then a major cause of death. Research in production of antisera to treat infection, and vaccines to prevent it, was centred in the schools of public health. It is strange now, looking back, why no scientist grasped the full significance of Ehrlich's discovery in 1906 of a chemical active against the causative micro-organism of syphilis; this presaged the whole modern development of chemotherapy in treatment of so many diseases, infectious and other. In 1920, however, the influenza pandemic was a vivid memory, and the epidemics of pneumonia struck every community at least once during the winter months. Children still suffered and died from measles, whooping cough, diphtheria, scarlet fever, and poliomyelitis. Typhoid fever was an important cause of death. It is, then, no wonder that the leaders in public health convinced the Rockefeller Foundation that creation of schools of public health would stimulate research, improve education, and advance the protection of the community from infectious disease by preventative measures. Education about maintenance of health and prevention of disease involved the public health movement in the fields of nutrition, environmental health (e.g., prevention of disease in industry), mental health, and health statistics. The public health physician or health officer was a most important member of every community, even in rural areas where this function was assumed by the general practitioner. In the cities, the public health officer became more and more a physician who had taken special courses at a medical school or at a school of hygiene. He was assisted in large communities by sanitary engineers, food inspectors, public health nurses, and others.

When one turns to that other, and to most people more important, health service, treatment of the sick, no advances had been made comparable to those in preventive medicine. The standard of medical care varied widely between rural and urban areas. Health services were rendered by the local physician in his office, or in the patient's home should he be unable to come to the office. Hospitals existed in cities and towns of varying size and were regarded by the community as a place where one had to go for surgical operations, very severe and usually terminal illness, and sometimes to have babies.

Sixty years after Florence Nightingale had cleaned them up, there remained the fear that the hospital was a place where one died, either because of the serious nature of the illness, or the treatment (surgical mainly), or what one might contract in the way of infection within the hospital. Mistrust of the hospital still persists in rural Canada even today, well over 100 years after St. Mary's Hospital was transformed by Florence Nightingale. Although country women will go to the hospital to have babies because the doctor refuses to deliver them at home, they often do not get in touch with the doctor until the arrival of the baby is imminent, being fearful that examination by the doctor may lead to complications (i.e., infection) at the time of delivery. Treatment, other than surgical, had not advanced for decades. Palliation of pain, and what was designated supportive therapy (maintaining the fluid balance, for example, and giving oxygen) was about all that could be offered the patient with serious illness, such as pneumonia. The physician still had need of his serious and knowing air of preoccupation that hopefully forestalled too-searching questions from relatives, who did not have the benefit in those days of short courses in medicine offered weekly and even daily by women's magazines and newspapers. Therefore, the anxious housewife usually did not know enough about treatment to criticize it, as she does today.

I remember my father during that era, engaged in general practice in a very small town, dispensing hope and encouragement – sympathy and consolation was part of his therapeutic armamentarium. His personality and the confidence it inspired undoubtedly supplied much of what the community sought in a physician. In addition, of course, he offered guidance in minor illnesses, set broken limbs, sewed up cuts, and assisted with the births of babies. All this was direct personal medical service, but he usually had another role in the community as well, acting as public health officer. This meant the annual examination of school children, principally of eyes, ears, and teeth, and vaccination against smallpox. He attempted to stop the spread of infectious disease through quarantine, and through control of public water supplies and, to a less extent, food. The general physician embodied the health service in toto, aided by the facilities of a hospital in some communities. In large cities individuals were beginning to appear who worked with the physician to extend his skills. For example, medical social workers were helping with the rehabilitation of the patient in his home and his community.

The nurse was still busily engaged in housekeeping: checking supplies of linen, rolling bandages, sterilizing instruments and linen, making beds, and bathing patients. In fact she did everything but sweep floors and wash dishes. Even in the operating room she was only permitted to hand instruments to the surgeon, expected to know by extra-sensory perception just what instrument would be required. Surgeons rarely talked in the operating room, the aura of divine power being easier to maintain in silence. It is so easy to forget, though, that the façade of omnipotence hid a bitter knowledge of the limitation of technique, and ignorance of why patients died in operating theatres. The physician, although the supreme arbiter of all forms of treatment and of every aspect of medical care, was pathetically ill-equipped by today's standards.

If one looks for indications in the 1920 era of the scientific advances to be achieved by 1970, some can be found. I have already mentioned the chemotherapy of syphilis. Today, chemotherapy includes organic compounds ranging from the antibiotics used in treating infections to those used in treating cancer. The hormones too must be included and especially insulin, discovered in 1922 by Banting and MacLeod with Best and Collip, in Toronto.

The momentum of scientific advance from the twenties to the fifties was slow at first, with the significance of the discovery of sulpha drugs and antibiotics in the 'thirties not fully appreciated until the intimate biochemical nature of their effect was revealed much later. During the Second World War intensive study of shock and its treatment resulted in a better understanding of its mechanisms. Then, when Bigelow cooled his patients before and during major surgical procedures to reduce shock and its complications, he initiated a whole new era in surgery. Of equal importance were the discoveries of new anaesthetics and relaxant drugs permitting prolonged anaesthesia without disastrous side effects. It is the enormous increase in understanding of homeostasis, the maintenance of equilibrium in fluid, and salts, and hormones and everything else in the bloodstream and body fluids that has made possible transplantation of organs, successful treatment of most severe heart attacks, and treatment of kidney failure.

If the sum total of scientific achievement in 1970 is measured against benefits to the community, however, the results are disappointing, because spectacular advances like heart transplant benefit so few.

To view the community of 1970 against the background of 1920, the changes are striking. Far more sophisticated than he used to be about health and disease, the average citizen now demands a high quality of medical care and is selective in seeking it. Furthermore, he has made it clear that health care is a right and not a privilege. He will look for it more often, and for less serious reasons than his grandfather. Today the individual with sudden and severe pain in the chest will call his general practitioner to get him a heart specialist, or have himself taken to the emergency department of a great general hospital. Normal women having normal babies want them delivered by an obstetrician with the highest qualification available, fellowship in the Royal College of Physicians and Surgeons of

Canada. They then seek a paediatrician with similar qualifications to advise on feeding the infant, and later to give the protective inoculations. The medical profession through producing more and more specialists has encouraged the public to use their services for the kind of care that could be given equally well by a general practitioner. The reason the specialists invaded the field of the general practitioner was that they could not earn a living from referred patients only.

When an individual is forced to his bed through illness, he expects to be treated in hospital. With grandmother in a home for the aged because there is no room for her in the apartment and with the wife working from 9 to 5 for five days a week, there is no one to look after a sick husband at home. Certainly, in the city, people have a different attitude toward the hospital than they used to have, and probably different from that of their fellow citizens in rural areas. They do not hesitate to go to the hospital for treatment of minor accidents or major illnesses in the emergency department. They may call their physician to meet them at the hospital, but are not concerned if they do not reach him. There are always doctors available in the big general hospitals, and there is reason to believe people with lesser complaints are seeking care in the emergency ward when it suits their convenience. For example, the peak load of patients in one central hospital in Toronto occurs between 5 PM and 9 PM. A pattern of medical service has evolved without plan. In smaller centres, and wherever available, such care may be based on a group practice or clinic that provides a wide range of services.

In the cities where everything moves faster, the public in its knowledge of medicine and its demands for service has far outstripped the doctors, who have failed to develop delivery of health care commensurate with public need.

In the far north of Canada, where government has played a major role in providing health services, 1 per cent of the population is spread over 40 per cent of the total area of the country. The semi-nomadic population is served by nursing stations and a very few hospitals and physicians. The difficulties of transportation even with airplanes, under severe climatic conditions, contrive to reduce the effectiveness of such services as are available. There is an excellent account of the services and the problems in the Report of the Royal Commission on Health Services.

It is evident that the health services available to the community today do not meet the demands of many of the citizens. Fewer and fewer general practitioners in the cities are available in the neighbourhood, and those that are have been forced by the pressure of their practice to restrict their services to certain hours or days. More of them are grouping together in clinics, with the objective of improving the service offered, and dividing the load more equitably. Hospitals, because of the mounting pressures on emergency and outpatient departments are developing general practitioner clinics. The trend is away from the individual, private-practice office for the general practitioner, and certainly for the average patient there is little hope for a home call by the physician, unless a relationship and reason for such personal service has been established previously.

To make up for the diminishing services of the general practitioner in the city, then, the general hospital is expanding ambulatory services, and city governments are expanding ambulance services. All this is to take care of those in immediate need of the services of a physician. There are, of course, other and important services in the community, based on the public health department, and assisted by voluntary agencies such as the Victorian Order of Nurses who make house calls and see that the orders of the physician are carried out, and, probably most important of all, teach the family how to take care of the sick. Well-baby clinics, mental health clinics, supervision of school children, all are encompassed by the health departments, as well as control of food and water through a host of sanitary inspectors of many kinds. More and more, the public health officer is an administrator with an ever-broadening area of responsibility. Although the public health officer is today usually a physician who has taken a postgraduate degree in public health administration, and is assisted by many other professional people such as the nurse, veterinarian, dentist, nutritionist, and educator in carrying out his manifold programmes in the community, he remains relatively isolated from the physician administering to the sick. The public health physician, oriented toward prevention of disease and protection of the community, has evolved into an administrator. He no longer renders service to the individual as he once did in the diagnosis and sequestering of infectious disease, but is concerned with programmes involving many people, or services such as food and water; his trained assistants directly administer the services. Naturally, the public health physician competent in administration of services protecting the health of the community cannot help but become involved in those services rendered to the sick. These often appear, and in fact often are, less efficient than the preventive services. It is the difference in kind and quality of service that often brings the organized public health officers into conflict with the practising physicians, ardent individualists resisting socialization through their political professional associations. There is today, then, a dichotomy in health service to the community, with personal health service rendered by the physician, and community preventive services administered by the public health officer.

There has been much discussion for some years now, of the health team headed by the practising physician. As discussed above, the public health officer has for years been assisted by well-organized auxiliary professionals, but the physician rendering personal service has resisted any delegation of his skills or authority. The result is that he performs many time-consuming tasks that could be undertaken by less-skilled individuals. His expertise is not fully exploited, but is dissipated by his intense attachment to the concept of the personal physician giving direct service to his patient. He will delegate responsibility only to graduate physicians in specialist training, accepting a supervisory role in that situation only. The result is that in teaching hospitals, direct control of patient care has now passed to the house physicians, and, while the quality of care is of the highest standard, the perpetuation of the system that excludes delegation except to another physician is assured.

The nurse, now escaping from her role as housekeeper, has not yet found her place. The physician has permitted her greater technical responsibility in the care of patients recovering from major operations, and even greater technical responsibility in the operating room. It is in relationship to personal medical care that the physician has not yet accepted the necessity of sharing and delegating some of his responsibility to the nurse. A diagnosis made, the average physician has not the time to discuss with the patient all its implications and the reasons and effects of therapy to be instituted. This the nurse could, and wants to, do.

Many health professionals, including clinical psychologists, speech therapists, physiotherapists, and others, are rejecting the dominance of the physician and seeking recognition as health practitioners in their own right. The physicians have not yet recognized that the only way to survive social revolution is to adapt to it, but adapt they must. Physicians are becoming more and more expensive to produce, and with the present pattern of medical education it is obvious that the medical schools will never produce enough physicians to meet the kind of service now expected by the community. The orientation of the medical schools is toward the production of medical scientists, necessitating selection for admission of candidates with proven intellectual capacity, otherwise they do not survive the scientific programme. Completion of a four-year university course must be followed by not less than one, and preferably two years supervised training in a hospital before entering general practice. But less than half of the graduates today enter general practice and of those that do, the majority have left within five years to specialize.

It is not surprising that medical faculties are pursuing research so vigorously. The biomedical field today is one of the most exciting sciences of all, where major discoveries are still being made. Nonetheless, the emphasis in medical courses has undoubtedly veered toward specialization and research, and away from the problems of health of the individual in his community. The crisis in medical research, expanding at an unprecedented rate, absorbing more and more skilled people, and costing astronomical sums, will soon be settled by government. At what point funds level off is still to be determined, but growth at the rate of 25 per cent per year cannot continue very long. As to the increasing number of specialists, they are quickly absorbed into the community, where many of them, in smaller communities at least, do give general medical care as well as practise their specialty. They do not, however, replace the general physician. For nearly twenty years now Canada has been relying on physicians immigrating from abroad to provide the general practitioners so greatly needed. Surely the present rate of influx of 400 per year cannot continue indefinitely, but it is the immigrant physicians who have manned the smaller hospitals as residents, settled in both small and large communities as general practitioners, and have thereby permitted the development of the great medical centres so oriented to the science of medicine. Without the foreign-trained physicians, the public would surely have demanded long ago a new approach to the delivery of medical care, and even, possibly, a new approach to medical education. While some medical centres in the United States have attempted to orient their educational programmes toward "comprehensive medicine," another name for general practice, the number of graduates entering such a career has steadily diminished. The trend toward specialization and increasing emphasis on the scientific aspects of medicine will continue. Canada is never going to produce enough physicians to provide the kind of personal service the community would like to have, because of the nature of medical education today, and the cost of producing medical graduates. The medical faculties are competing for that small percentage of students with superior intellect oriented to science, having already eliminated those with a bent to the humanities by insistence on achievement in physics, chemistry, and mathematics.

One is led to the conclusion that someone other than the physician will have to provide some of the health care for the individual in need of attention. This raises two questions: first, what is the role of the physician, and second, who will render the service? Obviously, one cannot dispense with the physician, nor will he as the most highly trained professional devoted to health care accept a secondary role. The objective should be to make optimum use of the very special skills only a physician has, which means relieving him of duties and tasks that could be carried out by people with less training. To do this requires the active co-operation that so far the physician has given only to other physicians in the hospital, or, in the isolated communities of Newfoundland, to specially trained nurses. It is just possible that at the present time the medical profession would be willing to support a study of the kind of functions they could delegate and of the kind of training required to fit an individual to undertake those functions. Obviously, the more supervision the physician can give, the more duties he can delegate. The physician then becomes the supervisor of one or more assistants working under him in rendering health care. As mentioned earlier, the concept of the health team has not caught on; yet the fault may be not the lack of co-operation of the physician, but the nature of the proposed team, usually considered to be the nurse, therapist, psychologist, nutritionist, and others. Each has a special skill independent of the physician, and is recognized as a health professional in his own right because of the skill that defines his discipline. None of these skills impinges upon the physician's duty to diagnose an illness, but these professionals do provide assistance in personal care, and in therapy prescribed by the physician. What I am proposing is the interposition of a professional who is capable of making simpler diagnoses and prescribing non-dangerous remedies, and who can provide a screening service so that only serious and complicated ailments are referred to the physician. One may well ask whether or not the sophisticated urban dweller would be willing to accept consultation and treatment with anyone less qualified than a general practitioner, but I think the answer is that he would. Today many people consult their pharmacist first and their doctor later, unless referred immediately by the pharmacist. Of course, the middle-aged man seized with a suffocating pain in his chest is still going to seek direct and immediate attention from a cardiologist, in a hospital. However, many, in fact most, ailments are minor, and most of them are emotional. One must face the question then of what kind of training and how long would be required for an assistant physician capable of making simple diagnoses, detecting emotional disturbance, and prescribing therapy, under the supervision of a physician. This remains to be learned, but some guidance may be taken from the course in Outpost Nursing at Dalhousie University, where experienced nurses learn enough in a one-year programme to be capable of providing good emergency and general medical care to the isolated communities of Newfoundland and Labrador. They have the advantage of two-way radio communication with a base hospital, and specialist service when needed. Surely, in less isolated communities the omnipresent telephone would permit the physician to retain supervision over his assistants.

There are tasks within his office, and within the hospital which a physician could delegate, for example, taking the patient's clinical history. Most physicians are poor managers, as shown by the way patients accumulate in their offices each day, by appointment, and still wait hours before being seen, but whether anyone as anarchistic as a physician in his reactions to any form of control would accept an office manager need not even be asked! The point that needs to be made, though, is that there has never been a study of the functions of the physician from the standpoint of what could be delegated to someone else, or, to look at the problem from the other point of view, of how maximum use could be made of the knowledge and special skills possessed only by the physician.

In discussing the future of health services the one real unanswered problem is who will render first-contact medical care in the community? and who will administer this service? One would hope and expect that the practising physician would not only supervise but also act as administrator of such a service, but to do so means taking steps at the present time to investigate the problem, to resolve it through training suitable people, and then to develop a pattern of delivery of health care that would succeed. This is the kind of organized concerted action that the practising physician finds so hard to undertake. His whole philosophy is based on direct personal service to his patient. He finds it difficult, if not impossible, to share that responsibility, except, as said before, with another physician, and administration is usually anathema to him. And yet, should the control of first-contact medical care pass to professionals other than the physician, one would be fearful for the maintenance of the quality of that care.

Despite criticisms voiced earlier about medical education and specialization, it is, I believe, apparent today that medical educators are convinced of the necessity of providing a curriculum and graduate training dedicated to producing general practitioners, or family practice physicians. No matter what kind of organization is projected or how many health professionals participate, the success of any health care system must in the last analysis depend on the quality and kind of medical knowledge that is its driving force. Such knowledge and the skills that must accompany it, are only possessed by the physician.

To support the physician in providing care, many health workers will be needed. I shall make no attempt to enumerate them, but would suggest that additional kinds of professionals will evolve, including possibly physician-assistants. Whether nursing will retain its broad range of activity, extending from the highly skilled technical role to that of specialized psychologist remains to be seen. One would hope that the nurse, with a long history of personal service to the individual, would continue to support a wide range of function, with specialization in the various areas remaining an integral part of nursing and not becoming separated into related but distinct professions. In other words, the basic education of the nurse should enable her, should she so wish, to specialize in one of several functions, such as intensive care, psychiatry, or administration, to name only a few of the choices that should be possible.

As the kind and number of health workers in Canada have grown over the years without establishing clear-cut roles and relationships with one another, so have the institutions providing health care. The active-treatment hospital has proliferated until Canada has more beds per population than the State of California, considered to be well endowed in every way. The cost of maintaining a patient in such a bed is incredibly high, and yet, in Toronto, the average length of stay in an active-treatment bed is longer than in most other centres in North America. The reason for the long stay, and thus the need for increasing numbers of active-treatment beds, is failure to provide enough accommodation for convalescent care, rehabilitation treatment, chronic care, and for diagnostic investigation. Each of these latter types of accommodation is much cheaper than the active-treatment bed.

In predicting the future of health services, then, one would hope that out of the present predominance of active-treatment hospitals would evolve a more rational balance of different kinds of institutions for health care, based as much as possible on small units, community oriented. The personnel would be related to the institutions required, and the range of services would include not only preventive care, but graded care for the sick and injured.

Initiative for development of a system of health care, including institutions, personnel, and range of service to be provided, will come from government to an increasing degree. Yet if the public leave all responsibility to government, there is danger of over-centralization of operation and control. What is needed to provide community support and pride of ownership is a board of trustees or committee of direction composed of lay people and some professional health workers, who would be charged with the responsibility of developing and controlling the kind of health care institutions and services needed in the community. I do not know what is the smallest sized community justifying such a board, but every effort should be made to break up the populations of the cities into units, hopefully neighbourhoods, that would support a degree of local government responsible for supplying the needs of the individual for health care, education, recreation, and social services. It is possible that such measures might aid in restoring to the individual a sense of place and purpose now lacking and resulting in so much mental illness.

Such trustees of health care services should probably operate at several levels, with representatives from the smallest community serving on boards of larger institutions such as general hospitals. The necessity for central planning on a province-wide basis is obvious, if there is to be provision of adequate health services throughout, but such planning will be improved if the voice of the people served is heard. The only way to achieve this is through participation of the public in the operation of the services in their neighbourhood, and being represented in the direction of larger institutions and services remote from their immediate environment, yet serving their needs. At present the Boards of Trustees of large general hospitals are primarily concerned with management, and expansion of services and beds provided by their institution. Relationship to other hospitals and services has not developed to the point where duplication of rarely used services will not occur. Regionalization of some types of medical care, such as heart transplantation must evolve because we cannot otherwise afford the cost in personnel and facilities.

If one accepts, then, the possibility of major change in the present facilities and services provided for health care, one must also be prepared to see such change instituted slowly over many years, because so much has been invested in urban areas in great general hospitals that have a long tradition of self-sufficiency in terms of providing active treatment services. Nonetheless, I do believe that by 2020, the people of this country will be much better provided for than they are today in the matter of services dedicated to maintaining the health and welfare of the individual. It is true that great advances will be made in organ transplantation, in treatment of cancer, and even in the prevention of heart disease, but these achievements will not have as much importance in the life and character of the community as readily available personal health service.

Having emphasized the role of the individual citizen in participating in the development of health care services, it follows that the basic unit providing such service must be in the neighbourhood or district in which the individual lives. I would call it a health centre, a place to go to with an ailment either minor or major, and also where preventive care such as inoculations against infections might be obtained. The staff of such a centre would vary according to the number of people in that community. Certainly it would have a nurse, a physician, a dentist, and possibly a pharmacist. Some would spend their full time in such a unit, while others such as a pharmacist and some specialist physicians might serve more than one centre. This would be the focal point for all the local health services available, including home care. One should not attempt to predict all the services that could be offered, because they may well vary from one district to another, and may be dependent on their relationship and proximity to hospitals. At this point I should make it clear that in my opinion the present concentration of casual and general medical care in the emergency and outpatient departments of great metropolitan hospitals is a misuse that has evolved through lack of any other means of gaining access to medical care.

The community centre must be integrated into a total health care system that will enable special services to be brought to the individual in need, or he must be taken to the place where the special service is available. Communications, and transportation of different types must be available. To indicate what is meant by communications there must be a system linking police, emergency treatment hospitals, fire department, ambulance services, and the health professionals needed in crises such as accidents and fires. Today in most major cities, police, ambulance service, and firemen are organized in a communications system designed to meet the crisis of disaster. Certainly their services are quickly available throughout metropolitan areas, but not in the more sparsely populated regions. Nor does the emergency service help the individual suffering an undramatic illness. It is to fill this need that the neighbourhood health centre must be developed, to provide service twenty-four hours a day. Sometimes, in the night, a telephone conversation will provide the reassurance so necessary to a mother with a new baby. Or, if necessary, a health worker could be dispatched to the home to assess the need for the services of a physician.

One tends to dwell on the necessity to provide help to those in need of treatment services, because today these are inadequate. Even today, through organization, and clear definition of roles of the various health workers, it is probable that a health-care treatment service meeting the demands of the public could be provided. Fifty years hence one would expect treatment services to be so well established as to be taken for granted. The emphasis would then be on health education and prevention of accidents and illness. This is an enormous field, and, although today education in hygiene and health is incorporated in the primary and secondary educational systems, one would hope it would have a greater role than it has now. Beyond this, continuing education in nutrition and in maintaining health should be one of the functions of the health centre, because the problems change with ageing. Health counselling, including mental health, must be available.

I would look upon the community health centre as an institution principally occupied with maintenance of health, but offering too treatment services in the home and within its own facilities for ambulant patients, and providing access, through its transportation-communications system, to specialized regional services such as general and special-treatment hospitals.

Outside the urban areas that are predicted to hold 70 to 80 per cent of the population in a few years, the solution to provision of health care lies in a highly developed communications-transportation system that will sometimes take patients to physicians or hospitals and sometimes will take health professionals to groups of rural dwellers, for example, to administer vaccines.

It is difficult to predict what the major problems of health care will be fifty years hence, when one considers that fifty years ago few would have foreseen the dramatic decline that has occurred in infectious disease. With increasing urbanization, increase in longevity, and increasing speed of transportation, it is probable that mental health, geriatrics, and accidents will be our principal concern. Personnel and institutions devoted to these problems will evolve, and, of course, so will the personnel trained to deal with them. Rehabilitation of the alienated, the ageing, and the injured will require proportionately a far greater number of health professionals than it does today. Care of the aged, for example, must not be regarded as social welfare, but as a problem of preventive medicine and rehabilitation.

It is my conviction that the real advances in provision of health services must occur in the service to the individual with emotional problems and minor illnesses, and help must be available to him where he works and where he lives. It is, after all, a very small percentage of the population that ever requires the sophisticated services and elaborate facilities of a metabolic or neurological investigation unit. Of equal importance to the treatment services in the neighbourhood, are the preventive and educational services that should be associated with them.

13
2020: Nursing fifty years hence

HELEN K. MUSSALLEM

Both the immediate and far-forward views are essential to an assessment of what nursing may become in fifty years, because the profession of nursing must always prepare for the future and yet practice in the present.

The practice of nursing in 2020 will be part of a total environment. Therefore, this presentation will first sketch very briefly the world of 2020 and the health problems of that era. Following this there will be a glimpse of nursing practice fifty years hence and the education for nursing practice in 2020.

It is known that many things in the world have changed radically and rapidly in the past half-century. The twentieth century has been characterized by unprecedented challenges to long-accepted concepts and by new, receding horizons of knowledge which, together, have created and motivated a social environment in which change has become an ever-present element. Now the rate of change is accelerating. This leads to the conclusion that the next fifty years will bring vastly greater changes in many areas of human activity. In broad, general terms, it is reasonable to assume that the work done, the methods and tools of doing work, the amount and the use of leisure time, the materials and facilities of the creature needs of warmth, food, and shelter will undergo tremendous evolution within the next half-century.

Certain aspects of the human condition will respond to these evolutionary processes. Demographic projections indicate that the population will have multiplied several times. In 1935 the world's population was 2000 million, and by 1975 it will have doubled to 4000 million. By 2012 it is estimated that the population will have doubled again to 8000 million. If this trend continues, the world population in 2050 will be 17,000 million.[1] In Canada alone, the population in 2020 will exceed 35 million.[2]

The present phase of history is likely to be known as the period when, under forced draught, western society intensified its educational processes and developed its intellectual capacity to understand and to use to better effect the chemical, physical, and mathematical properties of our world. The prospect is for an increasingly better-educated society, which, significantly, includes both the nurse and the patient. From this advancing knowledge will emerge a plethora of developments which will affect the environment in which we live.

It is axiomatic that from advancing knowledge will emerge further technology and techniques for doing work faster, more easily, and more effectively. This will influence the size and location of industrial complexes. The industrial complex will, in turn, determine the location and nature of the social structure and the environment of the segments of society which draw their economic support from this source. In principle, the by-products of advancing technical knowledge would be more leisure, faster and farther-ranging transportation, and better food and materials for use by society.

Since the population is increasing, and land conveniently close to industrial centres is not, it is difficult to escape the conclusion that large segments of the population will live, to an increasing extent, in high-density population areas where an effort will be made to provide the necessities for leisure as well as convenient opportunities for productive employment. This trend, which appears irreversible, will affect the environment in which most members of the health team will operate.

The preoccupation with speedy methods of travel of the past half-century will probably not have much effect on the trend toward the concentration of population into communities which offer employment opportunities as well as other necessities of life. Certainly, transportation by air, land, and water can and probably will increase in speed and convenience. More people will travel in response to business necessity, available leisure time, and improved economics. Space travel will indubitably advance our knowledge of the universe in which we live, but it will take an insignificant percentage of people away from their normal environment. And, although the nurse too will be involved in all forms of travel, the vast percentage of nursing will continue to be carried on in heavily populated centres.

In medical science within the next thirty years – up to the year 2020 – there will be spectacular advances. There will be more and a greater variety of organ transplants from human donors. The greatest strides, however, in replacing damaged tissue and organs to prolong life will be made in synthetic or electronic prosthesis. There will be readily and universally available, inexpensive and simplified human fertility control. Further advances will be made in computerized interpretation of medical symptoms, use of electronic prosthesis (for example, radar for the blind), and widely accepted use of personality-changing drugs. There will be general immunization against presently known viral and bacterial diseases by biochemicals.

During the same time, man will have developed an economical method for desalination of sea water. Automatic self-editing language translators with a capacity for correcting grammar will break down many language barriers and contribute to better communications. There will be new, ultra-light, synthetic materials for building construction, reliable long-range weather forecasts, nation-wide or international data storage with wide access for information retrieval, widespread use of sophisticated teaching machines, and automated libraries with the capacity to obtain and reproduce information.

Mechanization, automation, or both will eliminate more than 50 per cent of the manual functions now performed in production work, office work, and services. Automatic decision-making will appear at many levels of management. The use of credit, with instantaneous credit-rating checks will replace most currency transactions. The pursuit of further education will become a respectable leisure pastime for everyone throughout the entire life span.

Rapid transit for single cars and groups will be entirely automated. There will be widespread use of robots' service (including household robots), space observatories, a permanent lunar base, and a new concept of the physical universe will emerge as man frees himself from earth-bound traditions. During this decade, the evolution of a universal language from automated communication will be witnessed.

There will be extensive use of the ocean's potential for food supply – particularly on the ocean floor. Man will have developed artificial albumen and synthetic protein for food. Space travel will be less of a novelty and space stations will be established. Nursing in the space age will accommodate itself to this environment.[3]

As the new twenty-first century begins, there will be chemical regulation of the ageing process to extend the life span by 25 to 50 years, computer-regulated food production ensuring a minimum intake for each person and electro-mechanical interaction between man and computer. A present source of current information – newspapers and magazines – will have yielded to the advances of technology. By 50 years hence, there will be education through direct information recording on the brain, some use of extra-sensory perception in communication, primitive control of gravity, a landing on Mars, Venus, or one of the moons of Jupiter, and a flight around Pluto.

These are a few of the changes which futurologists predict for the years ahead. Inevitably, there will be a time lag between the development of these capabilities and their broad application to major segments of national and world populations, but all apparently are feasible and will exercise an influence on the environment in which the nurse will work.

NURSING PRACTICE IN THE HEALTH ENVIRONMENT OF 2020

What will be the state of health of the Canadian people in 2020? What disease will be "captain of the men of death"? What health problems will face the health professionals? Based on present information and trends, authorities indicate that it is not unreasonable to expect, from extensive research now being undertaken, a breakthrough in cancer, and there are prospects of controlling the great killers of today (diseases of the heart and blood vessels). Research will throw light on the process of ageing so that at the beginning of the twenty-first century more people will live longer. There will be less physical sickness, bigger populations, and less food. Complex living in a rapidly changing technological society will increase mental illness and the severity of accidents. There will be larger cities and less green space, and medical advances far beyond our present conceptions.

There is, however, one area in which it is difficult to predict any drastic change, that is, human nature itself – and in a large measure the work of the nurse is inseparably involved with the consequences of human nature. There is strong evidence in the saga of the human race to support this conclusion. At different times and places in history, large segments of the human race have been subject to catastrophic changes in circumstances of life. They have been decimated by wars, plagues, famines, and floods. Time and again, the survivors have lost all their material possessions. But, from each massacre and misery, the human being has emerged as just that – a human being with all the traditional attributes of human nature intact. There is little evidence to suggest that any change in the material aspects of human affairs, however revolutionary, will induce any marked change in the nature of man in the next 50 years. In the year 2020, *Homo sapiens* will be much as he is now, a creature of reason, who is born once, dies once, and in the interval between birth and death will be subject to most, if not all, the conditions and motivations that have applied to man since he first walked this earth. He will possess and exercise the capacity for love and hate, for fear and courage, for greed and generosity. He will be happy and depressed. He will be lonely, fearful, gregarious, and brave. He will feel pain when injured, anger when abused, and pleasure when pleased. He will, in fact, be the same human being of blood, flesh, and bones whose well-being and recovery from injury and illness now commands the time and dedication of more than 120,000 professional nurses in Canada. And he will respond then as now to the tender care and skilled competence the professional nurse contributes to the world of health.

The role of nursing will change as the health goals and the world of health changes. Nursing in 2020 is an exciting prospect. The methods, the tools, the materials, and the knowledge on which their development and application are based will be revolutionized. Inevitably, the practice of nursing must and will change with these changes in the nurse's environment. Within the context of a changing environment are found the stimulation, challenges, and opportunities of the nursing profession. These changes will be profound indeed, and the immediate and enduring role of nursing is to prepare for them, and to be able to function competently when they arrive – in fact, to be ready when needed.

The nurse has a triple role in life. She is part of the social structure, a member of the health team, and, in the ultimate exercise of her professional responsibilities, an individual alone with a patient. This will continue, and, particularly in respect to the nurse-patient relationship, it is possible to estimate and visualize some of the developments that will affect her profession, her work, and the satisfaction she will derive from it.

What will be the role of the professional nurse in 2020? This will depend in a large measure on how health services will be offered 50 years hence. Who will provide them? How many professionals and non-professionals will be involved? What will be provided? Why will they be provided? The answer to the last question is too obvious to require extended comment. All evidence points to the fact that although more knowledge and facilities will be available to help people maintain a state of health – as defined by the World Health Organization – the human being will still suffer from interruptions in normal living.

Many of today's health problems will disappear by 2020, as families will become more responsible for their own personal health through better health supervision and dissemination of health information. Progress will have been made toward the reconciliation of the great paradox of the 1960s which encompasses an enormous gap between scientific knowledge and skills and their application, for organizational, financial, or other reasons, to the needs of man. This gap will narrow, but as long as knowledge continues to advance it will never be closed.

By whom will the health services be provided? History is helpful here. At the turn of the twentieth century, there were three categories of health professionals – physicians, nurses, and dentists. Since that time there has been a phenomenal increase in the categories of workers within the health occupation. Although no precise information exists in Canada, the United States Department of Labor "Health Careers Guidebook" identifies approximately 200 health career opportunities, categorized into 35 fields. Statistics on hospital workers in Canada suggests that an impressive, though not as large, number of health careers are available here. This trend toward a proliferation of workers in the health occupation will probably continue. To avoid chaos and dissipation of health manpower, as well as costly duplication of services, the efforts to develop a co-ordinated and efficient approach in offering health services will be intensified.

In 2020, the physician and the nurse will continue to be the two essential health practitioners in maintaining health of individuals and, when there is an interruption in health, in assisting the patient's return to normal living. One impact of a changing society in the past 50 years has been a refinement of the old professions (medicine and nursing) along specialized lines, as well as the formation of new social institutions with their own professional specialists. Social work is an example of the latter development. But the essential professionals in health care will be the physician and the nurse.

In addition to the nurse, the physician, the patient, and his family, health care responsibilities will go to certain members of the health team, varying according to the patient problem. In the case of a school child suffering from malnutrition, the team would consist of the school nurse, the physician, the nutritionist, the patient, and her family.

Where and when will health services be offered? Basic health care will be provided by nurses twenty-four hours a day. "In fact," states Henderson, "of all medical services, nursing is the only one that might be called continuous."[4] "Where" is a more complex question. In the present patchwork of organizational confusion within the health field, it is not always clear to whom a sick person should turn as a source of primary care, nor is it clear to whom an individual should turn to find a consultant or interpreter to maintain health through the best that contemporary medicine has to offer. This situation will, of necessity, be clarified and streamlined. By 2020, the relation between the hospital and the home will be more closely integrated, with the nurse as the health practitioner moving freely between the two settings and providing a unifying link between the two.

The health-care institutions of 2020 will be heavily consumer-dominated and will bear little resemblance to those of today. In the main, the clientele in the second half of the twentieth century have been dissatisfied with the delivery of services by health institutions in a continual state of crisis. In response to general inadequacies of hospitals and referral systems, new concepts will be developed. Contemporary authorities believe that there should be six types of personal health services which can be provided appropriately by either university medical centres or by large sophisticated medical centres.[5] These are centres for tertiary medical care or superspecialty service, secondary medical care or consultant and diagnostic service, primary medical care service, emergency care or emergency service, social rehabilitation or neighbourhood health service, and a multiphasic screening service.[6] This classification of centres might well be used in 2020, although not all urban or remote centres would have all these services. The number and combination of facilities would vary according to the needs of the population and the facilities for transit of patients, clients, and diagnostic information. All these centres would provide health services, education of health practitioners, and research.

A spectre that will haunt nursing for many years is the dehumanized atmosphere to which advanced technology in these centres may lead. The personnel will work with highly technical "tools," and the care of patients or clients from admission to discharge will be completely revolutionized by the use of time-saving electronic equipment. No one predicts that there will be a "warm computer" to provide emotional support to the frightened, confused, or "normal" person. It is here, as all through the centuries past, that nurses will assume responsibility for the patient's environment, providing support, comfort, and highly skilled nursing care. The nurse will still maintain her unique, essential function, "to assist the individual, sick or well, in the performance of those activities contributing to health or its recovery ... that he would perform unaided if he had the necessary strength, will, and knowledge. And to do this in such a way as to help him gain independence as rapidly as possible."[7] However, her activities will change as the community and its health needs change.

To keep abreast of accumulating knowledge in the next 50 years will require increasing specialization and larger numbers of specialists. The population of Canada will have increased; the demand for health services will have increased; and, of necessity, the amount of work for those in the health field will also have increased. New machines, both for communication and treatment, will be highly developed. These will demand new organizational developments within the health field. There will be more to know than one person can know. More skills will be required than one person can master. It will be necessary to provide health care in many places at once. There can only be one type of solution for this sequence: a more creative division of responsibility and more delegation of accountability. This will inevitably change the role of the doctor and the role of the nurse. In looking into the future, it appears inevitable that circumstances will require the delegation of greater responsibility and greater accountability to better-educated nurses. Such a course is highly logical, particularly in view of the high specialization and changing patterns of practice in the medical field.

White states that "a strong case can be made for the fact that the solo practice of medicine by physicians ... is antiquated; it is certainly wasteful and may be dangerous."[8] In addition, medical educators

reveal that fewer and fewer recent medical school graduates con-
template general practice.[9] McCreary states that, "Increased demands for family health care combined with a decrease in the
number of general practitioners is leading to 'serious difficulty' in
the pattern of health care. ... There are progressively fewer family
doctors to meet increased demands caused mainly by modern health
plans."[10] If this trend continues – and there is substantial evidence
that it will – a more creative division of responsibility will be inevitable. Within such a division, and in the absence of other available
professionals, the nurse will become the primary person responsible
for the co-ordination of health services in the community and
hospital.

Brown's foreword in *The Coming Revolution in Medicine*[11] points
out that "... answers will not come merely from finding more doctors
and nurses but rather from a comprehensive review of the whole
domain of health care leading to the interweaving of new skills, new
technology, and new managerial methodologies into the total fabric.
It will call for the building of new paths for the exchange of knowledge ..." and the seeking of common denominators for the foundations upon which to build new structures of knowledge and skills in
health services.

Over the past half-century, medical scientists have changed the
course of the natural history of disease. They have learned to allevi-
ate suffering, to prevent crippling, and to postpone untimely death.
But current evidence reveals that this scientific knowledge has not
been applied to the needs of man to the greatest possible extent. New
methodologies must be developed to give meaning and validity to
advancing scientific information. Here, nurses, working in partner-
ship with other health professionals, can develop foundations on
which to build new concepts for delivery of health services.

Nursing is an essential component in any health service. It is an
art and a science applied to individuals in sickness and health. The
body of scientific knowledge of nursing is derived from and based on
the principles of the behavioural, biological, and physical sciences.
Its art is derived from the skilful and creative use of scientific knowledge and is applied for human comfort and welfare. This application
makes nursing a dynamic profession – always new, always changing,
always progressing.

Nursing is concerned with helping people to clarify their health
goals and, when ill, to help them identify their own goals so that they
can return more quickly to normal living. To do this, Hall indicates,

"The nurse listens to the patient, makes selections based on her knowledge of human behavioral sciences and invites the patient to explore them."[12] Nurses of the future will be more fully concerned with total individual health care. The present hierarchy of nurses in health institutions – hospitals and health agencies – will not exist in 2020 but the number and variety of practising nurses will continue to respond to the needs and facilities of different communities.

In the leadership position will be the nurse practitioner having the most advanced academic preparation, experience, and work record. She will function in the hospital and community as a health co-ordinator with other disciplines. She will be the family's health practitioner, responsible for their well-being in home and hospital. She will move freely from home to hospital, and back, as her services are required. Her relationship with the family group within her jurisdiction will be such that the individual will always know who "my nurse" is. Working with the nurse health co-ordinator will be three other types of nurses – the clinical nurse specialist, the nurse generalist, and a technical assistant. All these, except the latter, will be prepared in the university setting.

The clinical nurse specialist will relate closely to the nurse co-ordinator from whom she will receive assignments. "Her activities will include making initial home visits for observation and assessment, determining what nursing or other professional intervention is needed, and initiating health-team action. She will move freely to design, instruct, and give care for home or institutionalized patients, and carry through with follow-up care. In addition, she may participate in ongoing research activities"[13] as will the senior nurse co-ordinator.

The beginning nurse practitioner graduating from the university programme will be a generalist and will function in both home and community, preparing and carrying out nursing care. She will work with the clinical nurse specialist in complex situations. She, too, will be involved in nursing research. Working with her and under her direction will be a number of technical assistants who will perform technical nursing functions in the home or hospital. There will also be a large number of volunteer workers who choose this field for their increased leisure-time activity. But the senior professional nurse will be responsible for the co-ordination of activities of these workers to achieve the health goals of the people. She will indeed be master in the "house of the interpreters."

The professional nurse, then, will be the primary community

contact person for family health. She will be responsible for the supervision of health care in domiciles within the towering urban centres. These massive settlements will provide residence accommodation and educational, recreational, and employment facilities. The buildings will be contained in a climate-controlled, pollution-free city. Similar, but less sophisticated communities, will be located throughout the rural and northern sections of Canada. When required, in remote areas, the nurse will be able to transfer patients requiring highly specialized care to a specialized urban centre, by air buses or perhaps rockets. She will be sending them – accompanied by a nurse or assistant, as required – to their destination by computer programming of their travel plans and they will travel at a speed of more than 2,000 miles per hour. She will also, if required, be able to communicate verbally and visually to health centres in the urbanized areas.

The nurse of the next century will be prepared to use, easily and intelligently, all the new technological advances. As the supervisor of family health in the community or hospital, the nurse will be the health visitor. In her rounds, she will be assisted by the newest technological advances. During a home visit she may, for example, detect some abnormal signs in a young child. She will pick up the telephone or its successor and describe to the computer the signs and symptoms she has observed. Using this information, the computer may then tell her what to prescribe, or may ask her for more information to complete the diagnosis in relation to recorded information before it will outline the required treatment.

Only when the nurse has doubts about the treatment prescribed or is confronted with a more complex medical situation, will she consult one of the busy, highly specialized medical practitioners. Probably he will be located in a modern health centre and will talk with the nurse by telephone, viewing the patient on the television screen. In these complex cases, the doctor will ask the computer to display on the television screen the symptoms and medical record of the child as well as the medical history of the family. From this information, he will give the nurse a medical decision.

The nurse will then prepare a total plan for the care of the child and the family's responsibilities, using the medical decision as part of the plan. This is but one of the many ways in which she will combine her nursing knowledge and skills with modern technology to improve health care in the community. But her essential role will not be replaced by new technology. Computers, television scanning, monitoring of vital signs and symptoms, and other technological "hardware" will extend her eyes, ears, and intellectual capacity. They will not replace, nor be used in place of, the physical presence of the nurse. They will not replace the reassuring touch of the hands of the nurse, her compassion, her "cooling hand on the fevered brow," the cuddling of a frightened child in a clinic, the teaching of a young mother in her home, or research into nursing to provide better and more highly skilled nursing care. They will, on the contrary, provide the nurse with more time so that she can perform the essential role that requires her to be with people.

All new technology will, in some measure, change the activities of all personnel in the health team. This will be accompanied by and probably led by different concepts of educational preparation.

EDUCATION FOR NURSING PRACTICE IN 2020

How and where will the nursing practitioners be educated in 2020? The educational institutions will have undergone some revolutionary changes, as a result of a changing social structure, advances in technology, and new concepts in educational science. Today, the educational system is changing more rapidly from pressures outside the teaching profession and evidence points toward even more "interference" from all sources. Authorities today point out that, although children a hundred years from now will in most respects resemble children of today, much more will be expected of them in achievement and responsibility. "The new race of children will be healthier, happier and freer; they will also learn much more with much less effort at much earlier ages."[14] Present research reveals that half the growth of intelligence takes place between birth and the age of four and the next 30 per cent between four and eight years. Between the ages of eight and seventeen, when most children attend school, the intelligence increases only about 20 per cent. Therefore, it seems reasonable that as significant break-throughs are realized in the teaching-learning process, the infants and children of 2020 will have learned or have available a great mass of information. The traditional elementary, secondary schools, and universities as we know them today will probably not exist. The intellectual needs of all ages from birth to death will be met through use of an entirely different teaching-learning process.

At present we are experiencing a phenomenal rate of growth in computer technology. In 2020, some of the teachers in general education and nursing will become educational scientists involved in research for continuous broadening and deepening of new information and concepts. They will be responsible for feeding this information to the computer programmers. Some of them may then become computer systems supervisors responsible for the quality of information banks of scientific knowledge. However, it is unlikely that all teaching and learning from the cradle to the grave will take place solely through the use of videotape, microstorage devices, and tape-recorders. There will be in all likelihood a teacher in some kind of environment to provide face-to-face communication with the students so that they may have the opportunity to reach their full potential. This will be in contrast to the present traditional role of the teacher who dominates the classroom setting. Instruction in the year 2020 will, because of the very nature of the world, be flexible. Students of all ages will learn at their own speed and pursue their own personal objectives with the opportunity to develop their own creative potential. Hence, the person will not necessarily be educated to meet community needs, but rather the community will be the environment in which the person develops his own talents, a situation offering advantages both to the community and to the individual.

How then will nurses be educated, and where? Disregarding the formal physical structure of educational institutions, nurses' education will be part of the general educational process of the year 2020. In that year the content of their education will be of a highly scientific (behavioural and biological) nature, since the pre-professional student will have more understanding of the medical and physical sciences than the graduate nurse of today. This pre-professional student, however, will have proportionately less knowledge of the behavioural sciences, which will constitute a large part of the professional content of her education.

At present, the selection of one career in the health profession usually precludes the student from changing that career; for example, a dental assistant to a dentist, unless he chooses to begin at the very start of the new educational programme. Ginzberg points out that: "A person's occupational choice is not a one-time decision but the cumulative result of many decisions over time. These decisions re-enforce each other until the occupational path open to an individual has been narrowly delineated."[15]

In a society with limited human resources in the health field, this compounds the problem. With changes in educational methods and the need to utilize health manpower fully, a more realistic and creative plan will evolve. "Can several of the health disciplines be related in an educational continuum to provide multiple points of exit to jobs and re-entry for further study preparatory to a higher level of functioning?" asks Kissick.[16] The weight of evidence says this can be done. However, the implementation of such a plan has the built-in problems of any major innovation. At one Canadian university where attempts are being made to introduce the concept of interprofessional integration of the health profession, McCreary reveals, "There are fears on the part of medical faculty members that the scientific content of their program will be diluted by teaching other than medical or dental students. There are fears on the part of allied health professionals that they will lose their identity and be swallowed up by the monstrous medical establishment."[17]

Yet, by the year 2020, the system of preparation among the health disciplines will "offset premature restriction or closure of occupational choice." The education will be approached as an interrelated whole rather than merely an agglomeration of disparate categories. To develop new educational programmes from the existing ones will be difficult – but it will be achieved through pressures from the public and the students. The "Theory-skill spectrum in the health field" proposed by Kinsinger[18] suggests a method of approach to developing educational programmes in the health field. He suggests a hierarchical continuum in which generalizable academic and experience equivalents are common to several levels of functioning.[19] The student, then, must master varying portions of knowledge and skill in depth and breadth. If the student chooses nursing, she will be involved, educationally, not only in the special area of nursing theory and skills, but in clusters of knowledge provided for other health workers.

Education in the health field, as for other fields in 2020, will be a continuous process. Specialization in each of the fields, such as nursing, will also take place at the post-basic level. This may be achieved through a variety of educational approaches – through work-study programmes, through intimate relationships between educational and service programmes, through independent study, and through other avenues.

Will this educational approach to selection of nursing as a career have an adverse effect on recruitment into nursing? This is a moot point. The social usefulness of the nurse will not diminish, but an educational system which allows for an easier upward mobility may have an adverse effect on the number of women remaining in nursing. Even today evidence suggests that a decreasing number of young women at junior matriculation levels enter schools of nursing.[20] This competition for recruits to professional nursing will continue at an accelerated rate. The present trend of recruitment can easily be correlated to the expanding opportunities for young women of professional capabilities. Trends indicate that more and more women will enter the medical profession in Canada.[21] By the year 2020, the larger percentage of physicians may be women. This may enhance the status of women, but it will do little for the profession of nursing, which will continue to compete with a growing range of professional occupations for recruits. Since nursing will continue to be a necessity in any competent society, the requirement of quantity may be met by elevating the status of nursing through desirable working conditions and job satisfaction.

In a world of variables, there is one other thing that is reasonably certain. If the profession of nursing is to continue as an essential profession in society, it is clear that general educational standards must be higher than they have been in the past. Airplanes are not of much value without aviators – and sophisticated health plans, using the electronic, automated, and nuclear equipment that will be available, will not be particularly beneficial to the patient unless the members of the health team are intellectually equipped to use them effectively. The same situation applies to the use of new and different forms of medication as increasing knowledge of physical and human chemistry makes them available. The struggle for improved education will probably never end, but the efforts of the past half-century in which the nursing profession has sought to have students broadly educated rather than narrowly trained will, long since, have been successful. The educational emphasis will be on education as a basis for adaptability with competence, rather than on methods and techniques. This inevitable trend toward improved education of nurses, taken together with the equally inevitable shortage of time and numbers of the senior medical physicians will, as noted earlier, bring about alterations and innovations in the roles of the physician and the nurse. The long-established sequence of responsibility and accountability will assert itself in this field as it has done in others.

Increased demands from the public will make it necessary for more and more physicians to become specialists and medical scientists. A logical trend is toward the greater use of better-prepared professional nurses who will gradually reach more elevated standards as the upward pressure for educational improvement continues, and as a sophisticated public demands an increasingly voluminous and effective health service.

NOTES

1 Theo Lässig, "Planning the Future," *Scala International* (Frankfurt/ Main, 1968), p. 42.

2 *Report of Royal Commission on Health Services*, vol. 1 (Ottawa, 1964), p. 788.

3 Doris Ann Peper and Vivien P. Corrado, "Space Age Nursing," *International Nursing Review* xv (1968): 368–76.

4 Virginia Henderson, *The Nature of Nursing* (Toronto, 1966), p. 17.

5 Kerr White, "Organization and Delivery of Personal Health Services," *Millbank Memorial Fund Quarterly* xLvi (January 1968): 245.

6 *Ibid.*, pp. 245–9.

7 Virginia Henderson, *Basic Principles of Nursing Care* (London, 1961), p. 3.

8 White, p. 238.

9 John McCreary, "The Future of Teaching Hospitals," *World Hospitals* iv (January 1968): 23–6.

10 "Health Care System Threatened," *Winnipeg Free Press* (14 May 1968), p. 16.

11 David Rutstein, *The Coming Revolution in Medicine* (Cambridge, Mass., 1967), p. vii.

12 "Nursing Today and Tomorrow," *New York State Nurse* xL (1968): 9.

13 Shirley Good, "The Changing Role of the Nurse," *World Medical Journal* (1969): 14.

14 Leonard Bertin, *Target 2067 – Canada's Second Century* (Toronto, 1968), p. 87.

15 E. Ginzberg et al., *The Optimistic Tradition of American Youth* (New York, 1964).

16 William L. Kissick, "Health Manpower in Transition," *Millbank Memorial Fund Quarterly* xLvi (January 1968): 82.

17 John F. McCreary, "The Health Team Approach to Medical Education," *Journal of the American Medical Association* ccvi (11 November 1968): 1557.

18 Robert E. Kinsinger, *Education for Health Technicians: An Overview* (American Association of Junior Colleges, 1965).

19 *Ibid.*

20 Helen Mussallem, "Manpower Problems in Nursing," *Canadian Nurse* Lxiii (August 1967): 26.

21 David Fish, "Medical Students in Canadian Universities," *Canadian Medical Association Journal* xcviii (13 April 1968): 717.

14
Nursing circa 2020

KATHLEEN M. PARKER

The title for this essay is based on two assumptions. The first is that a nuclear holocaust will not have demolished all or much of the world as we know it. The second is that nursing will continue to be an important component of the health services for the people.

The history of nursing is shrouded in the mists of antiquity; its future, in the clouds. Practitioners of nursing in the twenty-first century will probably look at nursing as it was in 1968 with as much incredulity as we of the present look back to Florence Nightingale's era.

The future is not a discrete period of time isolated from the present. What our world will be in the early years of the next century is perhaps more a problem of control and anticipation than of prediction. Planning begins in the present for what we would like to see in the future, but it must be a flexible ongoing process. What we want now will not necessarily meet the needs of future generations or take into account unforeseen circumstances such as natural calamities.

CANADA

What will our world be like? The Commission on the Year 2000, organized by the American Academy of Arts and Sciences, has made some interesting forecasts. Although predicting the decline of Canada to an intermediate power, the Commission did not include this country as one of the new additions to the United States. Canada will be among the postindustrial nations with an estimated population of forty million,

In this postindustrial society, the per capita income will be more than double that of the mass-consumption society that emerged after the Second World War. Continued urbanization and the growth of megalopoli will result in a decline in the importance of primary and secondary occupations. "Economic" activities will be tertiary or quarternary. "A tertiary occupation is a service rendered mostly to primary and secondary occupations. Quaternary occupations render services mostly to tertiary occupations or to one another."[1] Quaternary occupations are concentrated in the government, the professions, and non-profit private groups. With a decreased emphasis on primary occupations, there will be less dependency on the availability of raw materials. Thus, the population will be more readily distributed across the nation. Advances in technology will make possible the "opening up" of the north for advanced civilization. Transportation will be so rapid and convenient that it will not matter where one lives.

The federal system of government will remain, although changes in its structure are presently being advocated. The central government will have to be strengthened to be truly national. There is a very definite trend toward socialism.

Technological advances are useful in themselves, but are more important in the changes they bring about, affecting all parts of society, especially the individual. Biomedical engineering will play an important role in increasing the possibilities of organ transplants, genetic modification, control of disease, and the prolongation of life through the control of ageing. The impact of the computer will be vast. An "intellectual technology" will replace the machine technology. Decisions may well be made by the computer rather than by a committee. Many new inventions will make life easier, for example, for the housewife. She may well have a robot "slave" to do her housework.

Existing goods and privileges will be available to everyone instead of the few. Sources of innovations will be intellectual institutions and research units, rather than industrial organizations.

The emphasis formerly placed on the rights and protection of property has been shifted gradually to the rights and needs of the individual. Will the use of high-speed digital computers be seen as an invasion of privacy? The present generation usually resents any interference in the private lives of individuals and thus reacts with hostility toward the possibilities of surveillance. Changes within

individuals and in their value systems may result in their being comfortable under such conditions. No matter what use is made of the
advanced technology, people will need to be educated to create,
maintain, and programme their computers.

Continuing education will be widespread with many innovations
in educational techniques. There will be a closer and more collaborative relationship between all levels of education. "... a variety of
new organizational forms linked more closely to community needs,
to work, and to living currents of industrial – political – intellectual
life than to the traditional community of scholars will be developed
within, outside, and beside the campus."[2] Computers will be used
for teaching and for providing comprehensive library references.
The development of communication techniques, such as television
via satellites, will enhance education as well as all aspects of life.

Not to be overlooked are the rapid developments in the past
decades of space-age probes. Even in this, the jet age, the ultimate in
excursions is probably a pleasure trip around the world. By 2020,
this may well be replaced by an interplanetary cruise.

This has been a brief look at some of the exciting possibilities for
the future. Where does nursing fit into this picture?

THE ROLE OF THE NURSE

The role of the nurse, in whatever activity she is engaged, is to provide improved nursing services for individuals. This, in its broadest
sense, pertains to efforts directed toward prevention of disease, to
nursing care of the ill, and to rehabilitation of the patient. The nurse
will fulfil her role in a variety of settings: as a nurse in one of several
community agencies, as a member of her professional organization,
and as a citizen of her community.

In the year 2020, the majority of nurses will still be employed
by hospitals (one of the community agencies). The role of the nurse
at the bedside will be to provide individualized total care.[3] To do so,
she will need to be skilful in establishing meaningful nurse-patient
relationships. While giving expert physical care, she will endeavour
to help the patient understand his condition and treatment. She will
also provide necessary explanations and support for family members.

Those nurses with preparation beyond the diploma level will

function in leadership roles at the bedside, in the community, in education, in administration, and in research.

Treatments and medications will still be important aspects in the "cure" of patients. Complex machines will assist the nurse to assess her patient's conditions more accurately and quickly. For example, routine use of automatic blood pressure recorders will allow her to provide uninterrupted periods of rest for seriously ill patients but still keep her informed of any changes. These so-called "technical" activities will be part of the total patient-centred care and not a primary function of the nurse.

As medical science advances, the role of the nurse becomes more demanding. Today this is illustrated by the care of patients receiving renal haemodialysis. The nurse in the renal unit has a considerable responsibility for the actual treatment. At the same time, she gives advice and counselling to the patient and family. Psychological support for these patients is of utmost importance while life is being maintained by a machine. Numerous questions are already arising in relation to organ transplants. In the future, transplants or artificial replacements will become more common. The nurse will have to deal with the problem of helping the patient to adjust his self-image to a form acceptable to him.

The nurse will work in a peer-colleague relationship with members of other health disciplines in either hospital or community. Dr. Rutstein sees the specially trained visiting nurse as the "emissary of the physician." "She will interpret the physician's instructions within the practical limitations of the patient's environment; reinforce health education of immediate applicability; administer prescribed injections or collect specimens for laboratory examination; identify new health and medical care problems; supply personal attention, reassurance, and comfort to the patient; and relay information back to the patient's physician."[4] All this she does and will continue to do, not as an emissary, but as a colleague.

In the previous remarks, "the nurse" has referred to either the diploma or the degree graduate depending on the specific situation and need. I do not expect the position of female nursing assistant to exist fifty years hence. If, in the next decade or so, the registered nursing assistants succeed in upgrading themselves, then the position of registered nurse (diploma graduate) will become obsolete. In the period of transition, I can foresee qualified persons among the registered nursing assistants becoming diploma graduates. There is also a trend toward preparing male registered nursing assistants, which is a highly commendable course. Although this may appear to be contradictory, I see these people as well-prepared orderlies. The title for this position would not refer to "nursing," once licensure was effected. An alternative course might be to have sufficient numbers of male nurses prepared at the diploma level. This could bring many other problems to light. Would the male nurse then request female assistants so that he could work on a female ward? Would he be assigned only to male units? If we are successful in attracting more young men into the profession, their interests will probably take them in directions to circumvent this particular problem.

PROFESSIONAL ORGANIZATION

By 2020, the Canadian Nurses' Association will represent all nurses throughout the country. For the benefit of nurses, it will co-ordinate nursing activities and will provide advice and guidance for nursing education and nursing service just as it does today, but with a stronger voice. The Association will license all those who practise as nurses in Canada, and maintain a national register. With similar standards of education in the provinces, nurses will be able to move more freely across the country. Already there is a move toward establishing a national test pool for registration examinations.

The national Association will delegate the administration of programmes to the provincial organizations. Funds for continuing education will be made available, if necessary, through the government and the Association. Graduate study will be sponsored to be taken wherever the student desires and a suitable course is available. Exchange visits for combined study and pleasure will be arranged anywhere in the world. The Association will also plan programmes for nurses coming to our country to visit or to work.

Members of the Association will scrutinize legislation introduced at all levels of government, watching for any points affecting nursing. There will be greater co-operation and less competition between vested interests. History was made in December 1967, with the first joint CNA-CMA-CHA Conference held in Montebello, Quebec. The Association will be responsible for evaluating nursing service within hospitals, with approval of the Association being included in the criteria for the accreditation of hospitals. Extension of the concept of accreditation to other agencies will maintain this relationship.

Legal counselling will still be available for groups and individuals.

Basic salaries will be established on a nationwide basis with recognition given for all types of post-basic education. Individual nurses will also be entitled to merit increases on the basis of quality nursing care. Research into nursing problems will be correlated at the national level so that duplication of studies will be avoided.

NURSING EDUCATION

At the present time, nursing education is in a state of transition. "There is a trend away from the three-year, hospital controlled diploma programs and toward the development of programs of two years' length in an educational system at the post-secondary level."[5] Thirty-eight years after the Weir report was issued, Canadian nurses can report only a trend. If we maintain that rate of progress, we will never implement recommendations for change in the system of preparing nurses. They will not be necessary because nursing as we know it will be non-existent. Nursing assistants will have usurped our positions.

However, there are optimistic signs. In March 1966, the Saskatchewan legislature passed an amendment to the Education Act which provided for the transfer of diploma nursing education programmes from the Department of Public Health to the Department of Education. A Board of Nursing Education will function in an advisory capacity to the Minister of Education. The new schools, to be developed on a regional basis, will be located in institutions conducting post–high-school programmes which have an emphasis on higher liberal education. The curriculum will be balanced between general education and nursing courses. Not only is Saskatchewan forging ahead in the field of nursing education, but at the same time a system of community colleges or similar institutions will have to be developed in which to locate the new nursing schools. The first such school was opened in September 1967 at the Saskatoon Institute of Applied Arts and Sciences.[6]

In Quebec, as an outcome of the Report of the Parent Commission on Education, schools of nursing will be incorporated in the general scheme of education under the Provincial Department of Education. The Collèges d'enseignement général et professionel are part of a new over-all educational programme for the province. Three pilot projects are currently under way.[7]

For New Brunswick, Dr. MacLaggan recommended the development of Institutes for Health Services. These were conceived of as post-secondary multipurpose educational institutions. Their purpose would be to provide semi-professional or technical health workers. "The NBARN is not satisfied with the disposition of its request for implementation of a new plan for nursing education and has asked to meet with the Minister of Health to clarify the government's position."[8]

Manitoba, Prince Edward Island, Newfoundland, and Nova Scotia also have looked or are looking at ways and means of improving diploma courses in nursing education. No definite action has been taken. In Alberta, two new diploma programmes are developing in junior colleges.

At the British Columbia Institute of Technology, the first two-year basic diploma programme was scheduled to begin last September. The course, a first in Canada, will offer common instruction to students in nursing and other medical technology options. "It is hoped that this will encourage mutual understanding and foster an atmosphere of harmony between nursing students and other workers in the health field."[9]

The feasibility of preparing a nurse in a shortened length of time was demonstrated at the Metropolitan School of Nursing, Windsor. In 1963, a two-year diploma programme was established at the Ryerson Institute of Technology on an experimental basis, with the evaluation to take place in five years. In the meantime, the Ontario Department of Health, with the reluctant co-operation of the College of Nurses, has introduced a programme of "regional schools." While independent of the service organization, they are still single-discipline institutions. Other programmes are being planned in conjunction with the newly developing Colleges of Applied Arts and Technology. It is to be hoped that the Regional Schools of Nursing already operating can also be incorporated into CAATS.

In her comprehensive report on nursing education to the Royal Commission on Health Services, Dr. Mussallem recommended that 25 per cent of graduate nurses be prepared at the degree level to provide future leadership for the profession. By 1970–71, seventeen Universities will be offering an integrated programme leading to the B.S.N. degree.[10]

Not to be overlooked are the programmes for the preparation of nursing assistants. With the introduction of the shortened course for diploma schools, it has been recommended that the nursing assistant programmes be phased out. There is only need for two categories of practitioners of nursing.

Such, then, is the basis at this time for making predictions for the future. I feel that if nursing gains a solid foothold in the general education system, it will rapidly progress across Canada. Financing has always been the major obstacle to implementing changes in nursing education. I expect in the future that education will be such a necessity for the maintenance of the country, that education, if not free, will be highly subsidized at the federal level in fifty years.

Thus, in 2020, the pattern for nursing education will depend greatly on the general education system. As mentioned previously, there will be a tremendous need for continuing education for large numbers of people, including nurses. Educators will be even more cognizant of the necessity for liberal education to balance the psychological effects of the computer age. Technology has possibilities of making education a fascinating experience. Imagine a classroom partitioned into semi-isolated booths, each containing a pair of head-phones, a typewriter keyboard, a television type screen, and a photo sensitive "light gun." These cubicles and those in other classrooms would be connected to a central computer. The student would communicate with the computer via the keyboard or the light gun and screen. The student receives information via the earphones or the screen. Students may be working on the same or different lessons. Each will progress at her own rate so that brighter students will not become bored and slower students will not be left behind. A teacher will be available to answer questions or clarify particular points.

There will also be greater utilization of known audio-visual aids. Procedures may be demonstrated by movies, such as some refinement of the split-screen technique so that three or four sequences would be in view at all times. An instructor could just point to significant activities. Television via satellites may provide actual illustrations of health problems, e.g., in life on the moon.

In her forecast for the year 2000, Margaret Mead sees girls as still being directed toward occupations related to "nurture, teaching, comforting, and curing."[11] It is to be hoped that she is right in her prophecy. A recruitment programme will have to start at least at a junior high-school level. Recruits for nursing would then be

channelled into programmes which would provide more of a foundation, at the senior high-school level, for their nursing course. They
will have two choices open to them – a two-year or a four-year programme. The two-year programme will be conducted in a post-
secondary school institution, and lead to a diploma. The four-year
course will be analogous to the present university programme in
nursing, culminating in a baccalaureate degree. The students in both
programmes will have the same basic educational qualifications. The
non-nursing content of the two-year programme will provide credits
toward further education if desired. The nursing courses, as being
advocated now, would be of the integrated type. The diploma graduate who showed ability and desire could, at a later date, go to
university for a further period (i.e., two years) to obtain her degree.
During this period, she would study more advanced social and biological sciences, clinical nursing, and teaching and administration in
nursing. I feel that two university years will allow sufficient time for
this, if adequate preparation is given, beginning at the high-school
level.

Both diploma and degree graduates are "generalists," although at
different levels. With increasing complexity of medical care, there
will be, as evidenced now, increasing need for short programmes to
increase their competency in a clinical specialty. These courses will
be approved by the professional organization but will be conducted
in the same framework as the diploma programmes. Minimal related
clinical experience will be required as the nurses will have just come
from working in the specialty area, i.e., orthopaedic nursing. These
students may be required to pay a minimal fee. Since education and
medical care will both be financed by the national government, and
the need for expert practitioners will be great, I expect every assistance will be provided to encourage graduate enrolment.

Beyond the baccalaureate degree will be an increasing number
of master's and doctoral programmes for those who are capable of
advancing farther.

NURSING SERVICE

"By the turn of the century, it [the hospital] will incorporate all preventive and curative personnel and services and will become the
centre for community health. But the new hospital centre will no

longer be self-centred. It will be carefully interrelated in a community-wide and regional hospital system to meet the total medical care needs of the individual and the community."[12] The supply of competent individuals to supply medical services will not be able to keep up with the demand. Resources will be conserved by strategic location and use of superspecialist services. There will be one completely staffed medical centre in each hospital district which will be interrelated with a series of satellite community hospitals.

Automation systems will allow for more efficient use of both doctors and highly educated nurses. Since automation will increase costs, the hospital will have to operate more efficiently by being open seven days per week. This will mean an increase in labour costs as more staff will be required. Further complications will arise from a shortened work week. Nurses and others have to be employed or on call twenty-four hours a day as many services to patients are personal and should not or cannot be automated. Nursing education will have to produce sufficient numbers of graduates to allow for duplication of staff.

The regional hospitals will be centres for community health. Located in these general hospitals will be: "specialty hospitals, facilities for the care of the broad spectrum of chronic illnesses including mental disease, a group practice unit, a clinical preventive unit, the local health department, and voluntary health agencies providing direct services to patients."[13] All of these units will require nursing service. Continuity of care will be effected more readily with the resources located together.

After a brief glance at where nursing service will be required, the problem becomes one of organization. At the unit level, there will be a unit manager (trained in administration), a secretary (if not completely replaced by automation), a clinical specialist, degree and diploma graduates, male assistants (if required), and porters. Thus, the nurses will not be responsible for non-nursing duties. With a high degree of automation, it may well be that one administrative assistant could manage two or even three units, depending on their size, with or even without a secretary on each one. Since there will still be times that patients will have to be transferred from one area to another within the hospital, porters will be required. There would be a collaborative relationship between nursing, medicine, and administration, beginning at the ward level and working upwards.

As clinical specialists will undoubtedly be in short supply, one may have to provide care for several units. Individual wards then might have two or three teams of nurses, each headed by an experienced degree graduate and possibly sharing a male assistant. Beyond the clinical specialists will be a minimum of levels. There will be a Director of Nursing with one associate director to assist her. They would relieve each other on days off. There would also be a sufficient number of assistants to have one on each of however many tours of duty there will be (probably four) and to provide relief for off-duty.

Clinical specialists will be on duty for the two periods approximating the present day and evening shifts. Possibly they would be on call for the remaining two shifts. The ratio of graduate nurses to patients will depend on the type of hospital and the unit. During future night periods, fewer nurses will be able to provide closer observation of their patients than at present, due to the assistance of automatic monitoring devices.

In the core medical centre, there will probably be several separate buildings involved, in which case, there will be several complete nursing departments as outlined. Division may be on the basis of geography, clinical specialty, or a combination of both. Over all will be one Director, at the level of an administrative assistant.

On the basis of a six-hour, four-day work week for individuals, yet maintaining the hospital or other agency at peak efficiency for twenty-four hours per day, seven days a week, the scheduling of off-duty time will become a complex operation. Nurses will be relieved of this headache by a computer which will be programmed by a specially trained technician. In view of the emphasis on specialization, I do not believe this rotation will be carried out on the basis of numbers of people within each category, so that nurses would be moved all about the hospital. For the benefit of the nurses and the patients, each unit would have its own rotation plan. Even the part-time nurses would always be assigned to the same area.

A similar hierarchical arrangement will operate in the public health agencies. Consultants will parallel clinical specialists and assistants. I expect that in the future, these agencies too will provide services on a twenty-four–hour day, seven-day–week basis. "It is also already evident that there will be an increasing market for in-service training in any enterprise that wishes to attract able graduates already accustomed in their schooling to accepting meritocratic judgments."[14] There will be one in-service co-ordinator for the whole organization. Responsibility for the programme for nursing will be delegated to a nursing in-service specialist. She will arrange programmes applicable to nursing only, as well as co-operate in the presentation of the over-all programme.

Having dealt with the mundane, let us now take a trip and make a few orbits in space. Major Pearl Tucker is the chief nurse of the Bioastronautical Operative Support Unit (BOSU) at Cape Kennedy. This unit is prepared to go into immediate operation should anything go wrong during the blast-off of a space shot. They are prepared with separate emergency units for each astronaut involved plus accommodation for ground casualties. Again at splash-down, they are equipped for any emergency. Her nurses have been trained to jump from a helicopter into the turbulent ocean to render care to an astronaut. Major Tucker says: "We will certainly prepare nurses to work in satellite hospitals orbiting in outer space."[15] She also foresees the possibility of orbital sanatoria or hotels where people would benefit from the effects of weightlessness. "As bioastronautics develops, the applications of its discoveries will change medical and nursing care and education as we know them today."[16]

CONCLUSION

The foregoing description of nursing in the society of 2020 may seem contradictory to the present influence of the ascending social sciences. A new wave of humanism has resulted in the emergence of a new psychology concerned with people, values, perceptions, and man's eternal search for being and becoming. New understandings about human behaviour and changing social needs promise new solutions to age-old problems. "No profession charged with responsibilities for human welfare will ever be the same, for, whenever our ideas about the nature of man change, great changes are called for in the ways we live and work with people."[17]

Throughout this work, the word "will" has been used extensively in connection with events leading up to the next century. To ensure that nursing survives as a respected profession in 2020, unity among members is essential now. This can come about only through a clear understanding by all, of "who" we are, "why" we are, and "where" we want to go. Significantly, the theme for the Canadian Nurses' Association diamond jubilee conference in Saskatoon in 1968 was "Identity and Destiny."

NOTES

1 Herman Kahn and Anthony J. Wiener, "A Framework for Speculation," *Daedalus* XCVI (Summer, 1967): 720.
2 Harold Orlans, "Educational and Scientific Institutions," *Daedalus* XCVI (Summer, 1967): 830.
3 Thora Kron, *Nursing Team Leadership* (Philadelphia, 1961), p. 4.
4 David D. Rutstein, "At the Turn of the Next Century," in *Hospitals, Doctors, and The Public Interest*, ed. John H. Knowles (Cambridge, Mass., 1965), p. 310.
5 News Item, *Canadian Nurse* LXIV (January 1968): 10.
6 Linda Long, "Tomorrow's nursing education in Saskatchewan," *Canadian Nurse* LXIII (April 1967): 30.
7 New Item, *Canadian Nurse* LXIV (January 1968): 11.
8 News Item, *Canadian Nurse* LXIII (August 1967): 11.
9 News Item, *Canadian Nurse* LXIII (May 1967): 12.
10 Helen M. Carpenter, "Nursing Education in Canada," *International Nursing Review* XIII (1966): 29.
11 Margaret Mead, "The Life Cycle and Its Variations," *Daedalus* XCVI (Summer, 1967): 873.
12 Rutstein, "At the Turn of the Next Century," p. 293.
13 *Ibid.*, p. 303.
14 David Riesman, "Notes on Meritocracy," *Daedalus* XCVI (Summer, 1967): 905.
15 Gloria Biggs, "The Stars Beckon: Report of an Interview with Major Pearl Tucker," *American Journal of Nursing* LXVII (1967): 1652.
16 *Ibid.*, p. 1653.
17 Arthur W. Combs, *The Professional Education of Teachers* (Boston, 1965), p. vi.

PART FOUR BIBLIOGRAPHY

Allemang, Margaret. "An Analysis of the Experiences of Eight Cardiac Patients During a Period of Hospitalization in a General Hospital," *The Canadian Nurse* LV (August 1959): 702–11.

——— *The Experience of Eight Cardiac Patients During a Period of Hospitalization in a General Hospital.* Toronto: University of Toronto, School of Nursing Alumni, 1960. P. 114.

Barter, Marion I. (née Tressider). "A Study of the Needs of Cancer Patients in Waterloo County." *Canadian Journal of Public Health* XLIX (November 1958): 470–80.

——— "The Pilot Home Care Programme of Toronto." *Canadian Journal of Public Health* LIV (February 1963): 55–62.

Barter, Marion I., and Ruane, Kathleen. *Continuing Education for Nurses: A Study of the Need for Continuing Education for Registered Nurses in Ontario.* Toronto: School of Nursing and Division of University Extension, 1969. P. iv + 63.

Burwell, Dorothy M. "Changing Attitudes and Images." *The Canadian Nurse* LX (February 1963): 122–5.

Burwell, Dorothy M. (née Dix). "Role Playing in Nursing Education." *Group Psychotherapy* XV (March 1962): 231–5.

——— "Psychodrama." *The Canadian Nurse* LXV (May 1969): 44–6.

Cahoon, Margaret C. "The Development of Empirical Guiding Principles and Criteria for School Health Programmes in Canada." Paper read before the Research Council, American School Health Association Annual Meeting, Detroit, Michigan, 9 November 1968. *Journal of School Health* XXXIX (December 1969).

Cahoon, Margaret C., Doyle, M. T., and McHendry, E. W. "The Consumption of Recommended Foods by Children in Relation to Sex, the Use of Sweet Foods, and Employment of Mothers." *Canadian Journal of Public Health* XLIV (July 1953): 259–62.

Cahoon, Margaret C., and Rhodes, A. J. "Health Education in Canada." *Health Education* II (March–April 1963): 2–8.

Carpenter, Helen M. "The Role of the Nurse in the Total Health Programme." *The Canadian Nurse* LIV (August 1957): 720–6.

—— *The Need for Assistance of Mothers with First Babies.* Toronto: University of Toronto School of Nursing Alumni, 1966. P. 99.

—— "Nursing Education in Canada." *International Nursing Review* XIII (September-October 1966): 29–35.

—— "Parent Education: The Need for Continuity of Care." *Medical Services Journal* XXIII (April 1967): 574–80.

Duncanson, M. Blanche. "The Nightingale School of Nursing, Toronto." *The Canadian Nurse* LVI (September 1960): 802–4.

—— "Who Speaks for Nurses and Nursing?" *The Canadian Nurse* LIX (July 1963): 615–21.

Emory, Florence H. M. *Public Health Nursing in Canada: Principles and Practice*, 2nd ed. Toronto: Macmillan Company of Canada, 1953. P. 397.

—— "Course in Public Health Nursing." *The Canadian Nurse* XXII (November 1926): 585–6.

—— "The University Department of Public Health Nursing." *The Canadian Nurse* XXVI (May 1930): 249–50.

—— "Yesterday and Tomorrow." *The Canadian Nurse* XXX (August 1934): 349–52.

—— "The University School of Nursing." *The Canadian Nurse* XXXIV (June 1938): 297–302.

—— "Nursing Service 1950." *The Canadian Nurse* XLVI (February 1950): 105–6.

—— "Preparation for Administration and Supervision in Public Health Nursing." *The Canadian Nurse* LXVII (June 1951): 418–20.

—— "The International Council of Nurses; A World Force in Nursing." *The Canadian Nurse* XLVI (September 1960): 713–20.

—— "Edith Kathleen Russell." *The International Nursing Review* XI (May-June 1964): 9–11.

Fidler, Nettie D. "The Preparation for Professional Nursing." *The Canadian Nurse* LX (September 1944): 621–6.

—— "Supply and Demand in Nursing." *Canadian Journal of Public Health* XXXVIII (November 1947): 509–14.

—— "The Metropolitan School of Nursing." *The Canadian Nurse* XLVIII (November 1952): 887–91.

—— "The Need for Research in Nursing." *The Canadian Nurse* LV (March 1959): 224–6.

Fidler, Nettie D., and Gray, Kenneth G. *Law and the Practice of Nursing*. Toronto: Ryerson Press, 1947. P. 106.

—— "Metropolitan School of Nursing Biennial Report." *The Canadian Nurse* XLVI (May 1950): 373–4.

—— "Post-Basic Nursing Education." *The International Nursing Review* V (January 1958): 6–10.

Hayward, Margaret (Phillips). "Correlates of Approval and Disapproval Received by Students at Selected Schools of Nursing." Unpublished Ph.D. dissertation, University of Pittsburgh, 1969. P. 119.

Hayward, Margaret (Phillips), and Dwyer, John H. "Students on a Children's Psychiatric Service." *American Journal of Nursing* LIV (August 1964): 94–7.

Johnson, Barbara A. (née Anderson), and Dumas, Rhetaugh G. "Psychological Preparation Beneficial if Based on Individual's Needs." *Hospital Topics* XLII (May 1964): 79.

Johnson, Barbara A. (née Anderson), Dumas, Rhetaugh G., and Leonard, Robert C. "The Importance of the Expressive Function in Preoperative Preparation." In *Social Interaction and Patient Care*, edited by James K. Skipper and Robert C. Leonard. Philadelphia: J. B. Lippincott Co., 1965. P. 16–29.

Johnson, Barbara A. (née Anderson), Johnson, Jean E., and Dumas, Rhetaugh G. "Interpersonal Relations: The Essence of Nursing Care." *Nursing Forum* VI (Summer 1967): 325–34.

Johnson, Barbara A. (née Anderson), and Leonard, Robert C. "The Nurse's Role in Individualizing the Admission Process in a Psychiatric Hospital." *The American Journal of Psychiatry* CXX (March, 1964): 890–3.

Johnson, Barbara A. (née Anderson), Mertz, Hilda, and Leonard, Robert C. "Two Experimental Tests of a Patient-Centered Admission Process." *Nursing Research* XIV (Spring 1965): 151–6.

Jones, Phyllis E. "The Public Health Nurse and General Practice." *The Canadian Nurse* LXIV (July, 1968): 43–4.

—— *Family Doctor-Public Health Nurse Teamwork. A Report of a Study*. Toronto: University of Toronto School of Nursing, 1969. P. 58.

—— "The East York Public Health Nursing Project." *Canadian Journal of Public Health* LX (June 1969): 242–6.

Jones, Phyllis E., and Bondy, Doreen M. "Family Health Service:

The Public Health Nurse and the General Practitioner." *The Canadian Nurse* LXV (September 1969): 38–40.

Parker, Nora I. *Graduates of the Basic Course, University of Toronto School of Nursing, 1946–1966.* Toronto: School of Nursing, 1968. P. 66.

―――― "Public Health Nursing Education and the Undergraduate Nurse." *The Canadian Nurse* XXII (November 1926): 563–8.

―――― "Canadian Universities and Canadian Schools of Nursing." *The Canadian Nurse* XXIV (December 1928): 627–30.

―――― "The Training of a Public Health Nurse." *The Canadian Nurse* XXV (February 1929): 78–82.

Russell, Edith Kathleen. "The Teaching of Public Health Nursing in The University of Toronto." Reprinted from *Methods and Problems of Medical Education.* Twenty-first series. New York: The Rockefeller Foundation, 1932. P. 6.

―――― "A New School of Nursing." *The Canadian Nurse* XXIX (June 1933): 285–90.

―――― "One Whole and Direct Training." *The Canadian Nurse* XXXIII (February 1937): 75–7.

―――― "The Philosophy of the Curriculum." *The Canadian Nurse* XXXIV (September 1938): 485–7.

―――― "The Proposed Curriculum in Action." *The Canadian Nurse* XXXIV (September 1938): 498–505.

―――― "Fifty Years of Medical Progress; Medicine as A Social Instrument: Nursing." *The New England Journal of Medicine* CCLXIV (March 1951): 439–45.

―――― *The Report of a Study of Nursing Education in New Brunswick.* Fredericton: University of New Brunswick, 1956. P. 76.

―――― "A Review of Nursing Education in New Brunswick." *Canadian Journal of Public Health* XLVIII (February 1957): 76–80.

―――― "Changes in the Patterns of Nursing." *The Canadian Nurse* LIV (June 1958): 529–32.

Russell, Edith Kathleen, and Wilson, M. Jean. "Nursing Education – Methods of Clinical Instruction." *The Canadian Nurse* XLV (November 1949): 820–5.

Wilson, M. Jean. "Clinical Teaching and Supervision." *The Canadian Nurse* XXXVIII (September 1942): 260–2.

Wright, Leora R. "Pre-School Programmes for the Mentally Retarded in Canada." *Mental Retardation* XIX (January 1969): 8–12.

Lightning Source UK Ltd.
Milton Keynes UK
UKHW020020210722
406167UK00009B/813

9 780802 061126